"There are many people who have felt compelled to write to Jillian since her first book was published. They have their own stories to share, stories filled with heartache, struggle, and frustration. In these selected stories, each individual found their way to an optometrist who provided them with vision therapy, which helped them finally find success. Jillian's enthusiasm and her happiness that others have found help through vision therapy is infectious. It is my sincere hope that everyone who struggles at school or work will read this book (and *Jillian's Story*) so that they too may seek out the care of a developmental optometrist and find out if vision therapy can help them."

—**David A. Damari**, OD, FCOVD, FAAO
Dean, Michigan College of Optometry at Ferris State University

"Jillian's first book was about her and the struggles she faced with her visual problems—seemingly alone. After the first book was published, she began to receive stories from all over the world about similar situations that were being addressed with vision therapy. The incidence is much more common than isolated incidents, and she was compelled to get that word out. She has opened that door in her second book so that others will not feel alone and isolated."

—**Glen T. Steele**, OD, FCOVD, FAAO
Professor of Pediatric Optometry, Southern College of Optometry, Memphis, Tennessee

"A marvelous book! It was a delight to read this book full of amazing success stories. Now we not only have *Jillian's Story* but also twenty-two more tales of vision therapy success to share with our patients. As a behavioral optometrist, I will be able to demonstrate to and motivate patients with the wonders of vision therapy. Muy bueno!"

—**Berenice Velázquez Sánchez**, MCB, LO, FCOVD
Optometrist, Querétaro, Mexico

"Deeply moving and important, *Dear Jillian* tells the stories of twenty-two individuals, each struggling with different injuries or disorders. One has suffered multiple strokes, another sustained a closed head injury, while others live with common childhood conditions such as amblyopia (lazy eye) and ADHD. What these individuals share, however, are the vision problems associated with their condition, which remain unrecognized and untreated until they consult a developmental or behavioral optometrist. Optometric vision therapy transforms their lives. This book is a testament to the importance of persistence and hard work, the powers of vision therapy, and the capacity to change at any age."

—**Susan R. Barry**, PhD
Professor of Biology and Neuroscience, Mount Holyoke College
Author of *Fixing My Gaze:*
A Scientist's Journey into Seeing in Three Dimensions

"Wow! What an incredible resource for people to share the success of vision therapy. I have been a vision therapist for more than eleven years, and I was Jillian's personal vision therapist. I continue to be inspired and overwhelmed by the positive and profound life changes that result from vision therapy. This accumulation of testimonials shows how vision therapy touches the lives of many people in a variety of situations. Please pass this book along to others; do not put it on a bookshelf. Someone you know needs to read this book! Way to go, Robin and Jillian. Thank you for providing such a valuable tool to continue to change lives and reach as many people as possible."

—**Lindsey Hebert**, BS, MA
Vision Therapist, Jacksonville, Florida

"This book is a must read for everyone, not just in the eye-care field—including optometrists, ophthalmologists, and the students and residents of both professions—but for everyone who deals with people of all ages who are not reaching their full potential in life. The primary purpose of the visual process is the direction of movement, and visual problems are problems of movement—movement of all sorts, from the classroom to sports. This book tells twenty-two separate stories of people who had their lives transformed by vision therapy. There are too many others who don't even know that their lives could be improved similarly. This book can help to change the world by helping those in need get the care they need."

—**Paul Alan Harris**, OD, FCOVD, FACBO, FAAO
Associate Professor, Southern College of Optometry,
Memphis, Tennessee

"We often have parents and patients who like to speak with graduates of our vision therapy programs in order to gain a more 'realistic perspective' about what to expect of a vision therapy program. *Dear Jillian* provides this and more with its collection of actual patient cases and their outcomes. *Dear Jillian* is a brilliant follow-up to *Jillian's Story: How Vision Therapy Changed My Daughter's Life* and allows readers to understand how optometric vision therapy can significantly change and improve a person's quality of life."

—**Jackie Powers**, OD
Norman, Oklahoma

Dear Jillian

Dear Jillian

Vision Therapy
Changed My Life Too

Robin Benoit
and
Jillian Benoit

Dear Jillian
Vision Therapy Changed My Life Too

Brown Books Small Press
16250 Knoll Trail Drive, Suite 205
Dallas, Texas 75248
www.BrownBooks.com
(972) 381-0009

A New Era in Publishing™

ISBN 978-1-61254-132-7
LCCN 2013943388

Printed in the United States
10 9 8 7 6 5 4 3 2 1

For more information or to contact the author, please go to
www.JilliansStory.com

For those who change the
lives of others for the better

Contents

Foreword

Dear Jillian,

Vision therapy laid a foundation for my life. It has made a tremendous impact on the success I had in school and have had as a professional athlete. In writing the foreword for this book, I'm pleased to join you in spreading around the world the message about optometric vision therapy.

After evaluating me, my grandfather, Dr. Robert L. Johnson, a behavioral optometrist, suggested that I begin vision therapy, which I started when I was nine years old. Like you, I did many routines that seemed liked exercises using special equipment. The one I remember most involved hitting a ball that swung from the ceiling. As I often say, there is definitely a connection between the vision therapy I did as a child and my performance on the football field. I think vision therapy helped me develop many skills I needed to succeed in sports, such as quick reaction time, eye-hand coordination, and visualization skills.

I am also very proud of and inspired by the work of my aunt, Dr. Stephanie Johnson-Brown. As a behavioral optometrist and the executive director of the Plano Child Development Center in Chicago, she has worked persistently to lead this not-for-profit vision clinic, founded by my grandfather in 1959, which continues to help children just like you. She has impacted the lives of countless children and adults by serving as their doctor and also through her many presentations about vision therapy.

Whether they have vision, hearing, or other sensory issues, people deserve the care they desperately need regardless of their income. I hope the message of this book will serve as an invitation for more doctors to become involved in community service projects aimed at informing and serving children and adults in need. I was already aware of the benefits vision therapy can offer to those who have had concussions; however, I was surprised to learn from the stories in this book that vision therapy can also be helpful in the rehabilitation of stroke victims and those who have suffered traumatic brain injuries. Jillian, I join you and your mom, Robin, in believing that people of all ages can be helped if only they know about vision therapy.

Sincerely,
Larry Fitzgerald
All-pro wide receiver, Arizona Cardinals

Preface

After *Jillian's Story: How Vision Therapy Changed My Daughter's Life* was published, someone asked me, "Where is your research data proving that vision therapy works?" My reply was that *I* am part of the data. I said that vision therapy is for people and only people can tell you if it works.

I am not a one-in-a-million case. Countless people of all ages have been through vision therapy, and it has changed their lives for the better. I hope this book will open the eyes of those who have rejected vision therapy. Thank you to everyone who wrote to me and shared their vision therapy success. You are the reason our book is titled *Dear Jillian*.

I went on a two-year tour of America's optometry colleges thanks to the Optometric Extension Program Foundation and HOYA. I spoke to thousands of students and faculty, in person or via Skype presentations, and told them, *"You may not offer vision therapy in your practice when you graduate, but please know what it is and what it can do. You hold the key to changing someone's life in your hand."*

I hope you will be inspired by the twenty-two wonderful people whose stories are shared in this book.

—Jillian Benoit, age fourteen

Acknowledgments

Dear Jillian would never have been written without many amazing and generous people.

Thank you to everyone who shared a story of vision therapy success with us. Your stories made us cry and cheer. We learned so much from you and truly believe your stories will change the lives of others.

We are tremendously grateful to the doctors and vision therapists of each patient who shared their insights and results. We truly admire you.

Thank you to the parents, teachers, and spouses of those described in this book. We could not have done this without your support and assistance.

Thank you to Brian and Annelise and our entire family for your words of encouragement, and to Kelin Kushin for sharing her wealth of knowledge.

Our heartfelt thanks to Milli Brown, Kathy Penny, and all the wonderful people at Brown Books Publishing Group. Milli, thank you for your continued support of our advocacy efforts. You and your dream team of professionals make writing a book such a fun and rewarding experience.

Robert

"I had never read a book for pleasure. Ever!"

He should have died when he was nineteen years old. After a horrible car accident, doctors were certain Robert would not survive. They told his parents to go to the funeral home to make final arrangements.

In Jewish culture, it's customary to bury loved ones the day after death. Every day for ten days, the doctors told Robert's parents to go to the funeral home. Then Robert's prognosis changed; doctors told Robert's parents that he would live but might be a vegetable. The doctors thought at best he would have very significant emotional difficulties due to the major frontal lobe injury he had sustained.

But Robert did not die. It took two years and more than twenty surgeries to overcome the facial, cranial, and traumatic brain injury he received in the crash. He needed many hours of sleep and slow recuperation over those two years to rebound from the six-foot, 118-pound patient he had become. He survived the endless cycle of being in the hospital, out of the hospital, recuperating at home, and back to the hospital again. But Robert didn't just survive; he has lived a truly amazing life.

Thinking back to his early childhood in the 1950s, Robert remembers how much he did not want to go to school. His mother forced him to go every morning and he easily recalls those days of "torture."

"I had problems in school. I remember feeling sick to my stomach, the terrifying feeling of having it be my turn to read in class. I couldn't read well at all. I hated it. I would lose my place and couldn't seem to comprehend what I read," he said.

His grades were poor, mostly Cs, Ds, and Fs. There were no special classes in his elementary school in those days. There was no extra help.

"I remember having yearly vision screenings in school. I was always 20/20. They only checked my sight in the distance. My parents never thought to take me to see a doctor about my vision. I was never diagnosed with learning disabilities, so there was nothing I could do except suffer and struggle through it," he said.

In middle school, Robert was put in a special class, but it was truly just a class for "kids that didn't fit into regular classes for a variety of reasons—mostly kids with behavior problems." He found himself in trouble often and sat through detention almost every day after school, but somehow he graduated from high school and managed to get into college.

"I didn't have goals in mind," he recalled. "I just went to college because that's what people did and it's what my parents expected of me. It was the early 1960s, and the Vietnam War was going on, and going to college was the popular thing to do because it helped you avoid the draft. There was a college nearby that had open enrollment. They accepted everybody; otherwise I would have never been accepted to any college. I had never made an A on anything ever in my life, not even one quiz or any test, but they accepted me into college."

The first semester of his college career he earned a 1.6 GPA. He was put on academic probation. "The second semester I got a 1.9 GPA and that was with me working as hard as I possibly could." He chose a biology major because he liked animals, especially marine animals, and he thought about being a marine biologist. "I never had big dreams," he said.

But even the dreams he didn't consider big or important were violently stolen from him the summer between his freshman and sophomore year in college. He was in a catastrophic one-vehicle accident. He was a passenger in a car when the driver fell asleep at the wheel and hit a tree. One of the passengers in the car was killed and Robert was critically injured. He broke all the bones in his face and skull and had damage to his brain.

"I should have died. My skull was fractured in three places and you could see my brain lying open. My poor parents were told to make funeral arrangements. It was a horror for them," he remembers.

But Robert survived and ultimately found his true calling in life.

Following the accident, Robert had constant double vision. His ophthalmologist prescribed sixteen diopters of vertical prism in his lenses. At the time, Robert was dating a woman who worked for a local optometrist, so he took his glasses prescription to the doctor. "The prism lenses worked well at giving me single vision," he said, "but it did nothing for my reading and learning problems."

The optometrist talked to Robert many times about the field of optometry and encouraged Robert to consider optometry school someday. They spoke about vision therapy, but Robert didn't pursue it at that time. He decided to go back to college and thought about a possible career in optometry.

College remained very difficult. Robert's grades improved slightly and he graduated from college with a 2.08 GPA. He applied to optometry schools and was rejected by all of them except one.

"The Los Angeles College of Optometry accepted me in 1970 because they had more openings than applicants," Robert explained. Today it is known as the Southern California College of Optometry and Robert said, "They would laugh at my application now."

"I remember a rejection letter I received from the dean of the Pennsylvania College of Optometry. He said I wasn't qualified and wrote, *Best of luck in any other career you choose* at the end of the letter. I was devastated."

Feeling very fortunate to have been accepted to one school, Robert moved from New York to Los Angeles to attend optometry school. The first year did not go very well. "I struggled and it was tough," he remembered. "But then things changed in my life—and all because of one field trip. We went to a pharmaceutical company that produced ophthalmic solutions."

"They had two speakers that day, but I only remember Dr. Donald Getz. He spoke passionately about vision therapy. He described it as fun, rewarding, and life changing for patients and I knew that was what I wanted to do. I wanted to do vision therapy," he added.

Robert met many optometrists in Southern California specializing in vision therapy such as Dr. Homer Hendrickson, Dr. Robert Wold, Dr. Ralph Schrock, and many others. After getting to know Dr. Schrock, Robert decided to pursue vision therapy for himself—as the patient, not the doctor. It had been five years since his car accident, and, although the prism lenses helped him, he still could not read very well.

With a little help from his optometry college classmates, Robert skipped school once a week and drove from Los Angeles to San Diego for vision therapy with Dr. Schrock. "I would do vision therapy with one of his vision therapists, observe Dr. Schrock working with other patients, do another vision therapy session, assist with patients, and do a third vision therapy session all in one day. Then I would have dinner with Dr. Schrock, sleep at his home and drive back to Los Angeles the next morning. I did this for ten months."

Robert also did vision therapy exercises at home. He didn't tell any of his professors what he was doing, only confiding in his friends. "Dr. Schrock never charged me a dime," he said. "He was an outstanding optometrist and an amazingly caring and generous man."

During Robert's vision therapy two major events occurred. First, the power in Robert's prism glasses decreased from sixteen diopters to two diopters, which is tremendous for a vertical deviation. The second major event was that Robert could read. "I wasn't losing my place, my comprehension went up dramatically, and I didn't have to read out loud to hear myself." His grades soared.

Robert graduated from the Los Angeles College of Optometry with honors. He won the award for best student in the area of visual training. He was accepted for a one-year residency in visual training at the State University of New York College of Optometry.

"After that year in New York, I decided to go back to California. I moved to San Diego and joined a practice with a true pioneer in behavioral optometry, Dr. Amorita Tregenza. She was the first president of the College of Optometrists in Vision Development (COVD). A number of years later, I went on to become president of COVD myself."

Robert remembers one very ironic moment. "While president of COVD, I had the pleasure of introducing many people making presentations. One of these presenters included the dean of the optometry school in Pennsylvania—the school that wished me best of luck in any other career I chose. Vision therapy changed my life, and now my goal is to change the lives of others."

Jillian's Words about Robert

"Awesome" is the word that comes to mind when I think of Dr. Sanet. He is a giant! I don't mean a Jack and the Beanstalk kind of giant. He is a giant in the world of optometry. Vision therapy changed his life, and he has changed the "life" of vision therapy. Robert's transformation from a teenager with traumatic brain injury to a leader in his field is an inspiration to me.

After working several years in his practice in San Diego, Robert decided to make a change. He loved working in the vision therapy room with patients so much that he decided to devote his life to working with kids, especially kids who were struggling in school.

One morning many years later, he thought, "I want to touch a million lives." Although he had a large number of people coming to see him in his practice, he knew he could never reach a million people in his office. He decided to sell his practice and began to lecture and teach other optometrists about vision therapy. Boy, am I glad he did!

One of the million lives he has touched through his teachings is mine. My optometrist during vision therapy was Dr. James Horning, who learned many things from Dr. Sanet. Dr. Horning said, "Whenever I get the opportunity to attend one of his lectures, I do."

I think Dr. Sanet has probably touched a million lives. He has helped so many kids and adults as their personal optometrist and now, through his seminars, has taught more than one thousand optometrists about vision therapy so that they can help others. He has worked with USA gold medal Olympic volleyball teams, professional football and baseball teams, and professional LPGA golfers.

He created the Sanet Vision Integrator (SVI), a computerized vision therapy program used in many vision training practices. I didn't use an SVI in vision therapy, but I had the chance to play on one while making a presentation in Utah.

While visiting the offices of Drs. Robin Price and Jarrod Davies in Provo, I saw this amazingly cool big screen TV on the wall in one of the vision therapy rooms. I blazed right over to it, excited to play some computer games. After playing for a few seconds, I said to Drs. Price and Davies, "Hey, this is like a Wii rotator!"

The rotator I used in vision therapy was a piece of machinery with a round pegboard that moved in a circle. I did my best to put golf tees in the holes called out by my vision therapist. But the SVI allows kids to do the same exercise while touching a computer screen. The SVI makes it fun, like a video game, but it's a great visual exercise as well.

I know I want to work in the field of vision therapy someday. When asked what advice he would give me, Dr. Sanet said, "Work hard. Believe in yourself. Have big dreams." One of his favorite sayings is, "The true gift of giving is planting trees under whose shade you will never sit."

From this young lady who was lucky enough to sit in the shade of a tree you planted, thank you, Dr. Sanet. You will always be my favorite giant!

Matthew

"When I said, 'Mom, I can see,' she started happy crying."

Matthew's parents remember an evening not too long ago when their son showed them a twelve-minute video on his iPad: a video of Matthew reading.

"My mom was sitting on the couch crying, but my dad didn't cry because he is brave," Matthew said. His dad, Jim, was quick to admit that he cried too.

"He read a book called *Sunny Weather Days* and my husband and I were in tears. We looked at each other wondering, *Where is this coming from? How in the world is he reading like that?*" said Matthew's mother, Pat. "He was sounding out words like *sunblock, shadow,* and even *weather,*" she said. "About an hour later it dawned on us: *his vision therapy, of course!* Then we really cried!"

This might not sound like a major accomplishment to some, but Matthew has Down syndrome. Through the years, Matthew's parents had pushed his schools to teach him to read, and he had some success with kindergarten-level reading skills. But even at the age of seventeen, he was still unable to sound out words or to read more advanced material.

Matthew was diagnosed with Down syndrome shortly after his birth. His parents did not know they were expecting a child with special needs. With three older children, they admitted that Matthew's challenges opened their eyes to a whole new world.

Matthew had surgery at the age of five to fuse his first three vertebrae to his skull due to Atlantoaxial instability. Doctors hoped the surgery would stabilize Matthew's neck, allowing him to play normally and safely. Without the surgery, he could easily break his neck and become paralyzed, even from a simple fall.

Then, at the age of ten, Matthew was diagnosed with acute lymphocytic leukemia. He had chemotherapy treatments for more than three years. "They did such a great job with Matthew at Doernbecher Children's Hospital in Portland, and he had such a great experience that he is always excited to go to the doctor," said Jim. "You'd think it would be the other way," he added.

Living more than 250 miles from Portland, Matthew and his parents spent many hours in the car going to doctors' appointments. "With all the travel, Matthew would usually have some in-car activities or a DVD to watch," said Jim. "We would point out a mountain or beautiful scenery, but he didn't act interested," he added.

On one trip to an appointment in Portland, Pat went to a workshop sponsored by the Special Olympics. "They were checking eyes and giving away glasses that day. Matthew was about eleven or twelve and when he put on the glasses he said, 'I can see,' and I started crying," Pat said.

Matthew had gone to an ophthalmologist numerous times growing up and he had never been diagnosed with a vision problem. Pat said, "I guess Matthew slipped through the cracks because of his limited communications skills, but the Special Olympics volunteers knew how to examine him in a way that identified his sight problem," she added.

Pat returned to the ophthalmologist's office when Matthew was about fifteen because she and Jim had noticed an eye turn. Pat shared,

"I asked the doctor if Matthew had a lazy eye and he said he didn't. He said Matthew could use that eye if he wanted to do so."

When Matthew was seventeen, Pat learned about an upcoming seminar on learning disabilities through their special needs support group. "I was faced with the hard choice of going to a memorial service for someone I knew or going to the seminar. I decided my friend would have wanted me to do what was best for Matthew, and I went to the seminar," she said.

Jim said, "She came home all excited about vision therapy. Pat said she felt as if the doctor was describing some of Matthew's behaviors, and she chatted with her after the seminar. We decided to take him for an evaluation after Pat explained to me what she had learned."

Matthew first met Dr. Gabby Marshall in July 2012. He was diagnosed with a "constant right esotropia (eye turning inward) and no measurable depth perception, despite fairly good sight in each eye. He was unable to maintain fixation or track an object."

Dr. Marshall said, "Matthew also displayed poor accommodative (focusing) ability, a common visual condition associated with Down syndrome." She added, "He was assessed for vision therapy, and it was discovered that he also showed struggles in auditory processing, laterality and directionality, visual discrimination and retained primitive reflexes."

"At Matthew's consultation, his prognosis was discussed at length with concerns over trying to discriminate what was due to his disability versus a trainable visual deficit. It was decided that there were many possible benefits from doing vision therapy including improved peripheral awareness and depth perception," she added.

His vision therapist, Tamie, said, "At Matthew's first session he walked into the office with a hunched posture, shoulders curled inward, head looking down, mouth open, walking with a stiff stride. His gaze was downward for almost all of this first session; thus, he had difficulty with eye contact."

Over the first month most of Matthew's vision therapy activities had to be modified because of his physical limitations. Tamie said, "While Matthew was pleasant to work with, he had a monotone demeanor about him for the first month."

"Around the fifth session we started seeing changes," Tamie shared. "Some were very small and might have gone unnoticed by many, but his parents and I were aware of things such as Matthew showing pride in demonstrating an activity at which he had worked diligently during our session."

Tamie reported that Matthew was holding his head up straighter and his body muscles were more relaxed in general. She said, "Though the eye stretches were a little uncomfortable and not his favorite, he endured."

About nine sessions into vision therapy, Matthew had a health scare. "We thought he might have leukemia again and we took him back to the hospital in Portland," Jim said.

"On that trip, the most amazing thing happened. As we were driving near Mt. Hood, Matthew said from the backseat, 'Awww, look at that mountain.' We couldn't believe he said that. He had never shown interest in anything outside while driving in the car. And, as we got closer to Portland, Matthew started pointing out airplanes in the sky. That just blew us away and the tears started flowing," Jim said.

Tami said, "Matthew was using his periphery! He has made many trips, but this was the first where he was aware that there was vision beyond the interior of the car. He told me he saw trees, cars, clouds, airplanes, and mountains. There were many images that filled up his brain."

Over the next few weeks, Matthew continued to achieve new skills. According to Tamie, "He caught his first of many bean bags from the pitch-back net, his marching was turning into skipping, he was using his eyes without head movement, and he was able to fuse and see depth."

"Best of all, he was joking, smiling and laughing. He had self esteem and was more comfortable in his world," she added. "At our next session, Matthew showed me the video he had made of himself alone in his room, reading a book about weather. Matthew said, "Mommy was crying when she saw my video reading, but she was not sad.""

According to Dr. Marshall, Matthew just needed the control to hold his eyes still long enough to actually "see" the words on the page. The foundation for this skill comes from opening up and using peripheral vision. "Matthew had the intelligence and desire for word knowledge; his physical eye movement skills just weren't on the same level," she shared.

Jillian's Words about Matthew

Matthew is now eighteen, and he likes to tell people that he is a man and show them the whiskers on his chin. He is a sweetheart.

I join his parents in being angry that his vision problems weren't figured out until he was seventeen. Thank goodness the Special Olympics offered the eye exams that got him into glasses in the first place.

Matthew goes to public school, but in high school the focus for special needs kids is on life skills and not academics. Pat said, "We have always helped him and worked with him on reading at home. Getting him to do it was like pulling nails. We were just so stunned when he started sounding out words and enjoyed reading."

Jim said, "This was one more affirmation for us that vision therapy works."

Matthew has been reading to his family quite a bit lately. He even read to his big sister, Anna, bringing tears to her eyes. Pat has been searching the library for Hi-Lo readers in subjects interesting to Matthew. His school has expressed willingness to support his new reading ability, but their life skills curriculum does not leave much time for reading instruction.

Tamie explained how vision therapy helped Matthew to read. She said, "We didn't teach him how to read but gave him the vision skills he needed to connect with his brain and utilize what he had already learned. So much credit goes to his parents for their diligence over the years," she added.

Tamie expressed her pride in Matthew's progress. "Now when I go out to the waiting room to greet Matthew he is relaxed, sitting up straight, mouth closed, smiling while he reads one of his favorite types of magazines about cars. Though reading well is almost always a goal for our vision therapy patients, for Matthew, it was a bonus."

Pat said that she's noticed a difference in her son's posture. He no longer sits two or three inches from the computer. He has always liked basketball, but his teachers have noticed that his skills have improved.

Matthew never complains when it's time to do his vision therapy exercises at home. "He is all in," said Pat. Matthew and his parents put in four-plus days a week on home activities. "It's a lot of work."

When asked what he thought about vision therapy, Matthew said, "It's fun with games. It's awesome." He also enjoys playing video games with his friends, and he loves to take his CD player outside and swing while he listens to music.

Matthew said he once showed Tamie how strong he is by flexing his arm muscles. He said Tamie told him that they could work together to make his eyes strong too.

At his sister's wedding earlier this year, Matthew gave a very sweet and appropriate toast. Now I hope to do the same for him: Here's to you, Matthew. I wish you all the happiness in the world, and I hope your life (in video game terms) keeps leveling up. You deserve the very best of everything. I'd love to play video games with you someday. And, to your parents, thank you for everything you have done for your son. I really, really admire you.

Teah

"There are many labels that can be mistakenly put on vision problems, and it just delays the proper diagnosis."
—Lizbeth, Teah's mother

Her teacher said she was lazy.

"Lazy would never be a word I'd use to describe Teah," said her mother, Lizbeth. "It's true that she had trouble learning to read in kindergarten. At the first grade parent-teacher conference, the teacher told me she was struggling, but she'd have to be two grades behind to get assistance," she added.

"Teah did well in preschool, but it started getting harder and harder for her as she got into kindergarten and first grade," Lizbeth said. "She was falling further and further behind her classmates and becoming so unhappy. She started saying she hated school, and I watched her literally retreat from learning—trying to hide in the back of the classroom, her head down on her desk, curled up as small as she could become in her chair, fidgeting and staring out of the windows. We felt so helpless," Lizbeth shared.

Teah's parents also noticed that she was not enjoying sports. "We signed her up for soccer when she was about five. I remember standing on the sidelines cheering for all the kids and shouting encouraging words to her about getting into the game and kicking the ball. She stood there looking miserable with all the other kids racing around her," Lizbeth remembered.

"My husband ran out to join the group and try to help make her more comfortable. She ended up hiding behind him and sobbing into his pant leg," Lizbeth recalled.

They took her back to soccer the next week, but things didn't get any better. "Finally, we gave up, thinking that perhaps she just didn't like team sports," she added. They found out later that Teah was seeing double from eight to twenty feet. "No wonder she didn't want to run at the ball!"

Lizbeth said, "My mother is an early childhood expert, and I asked her about Teah's struggles. She said to start with a doctor to rule out a medical problem. We saw our pediatrician and she referred us to our ophthalmologist."

Teah had already seen the same ophthalmologist when she was three years old for a routine eye exam as recommended by her preschool. His response upon examining Teah again really took Lizbeth by surprise.

"He turned around and looked at me after evaluating Teah. He pointed his finger at me and said that this was serious and he blamed me for not bringing her in earlier. I just sat there in shock. He'd seen her before and he was blaming me," Lizbeth remembered.

Teah was given a prescription for eyeglasses and immediately began patching. She wore a patch over her stronger eye to encourage the weaker one to work. She started out wearing the patch eleven hours a day and was later reduced to eight and then to seven hours.

"She was a good patch wearer because we basically bribed her to wear them," said Lizbeth. If Teah wore her eye patch as recommended, she could have a new My Little Pony toy once a week. Teah's parents recently gave away her My Little Pony collection to a little neighbor girl. She inherited forty-five ponies!

Despite the fact that Teah wore her patch, she still could not read. Lizbeth said, "After almost a year the doctor told me that Teah was close to 20/20 vision and his job was done. When I suggested there might be further problems because she had headaches and still couldn't read, he pointed his finger in my face and told me, 'You go back to the school and tell them it's an education problem.'"

Lizbeth shared their struggles with a friend who told her about Parents Active in Vision Education (PAVE), an organization dedicated to helping parents and teachers of children with undiagnosed vision problems.

"I went to the PAVE website and found a checklist to help you figure out if your child might have vision problems. I cried as I kept checking box after box," Lizbeth said.

Teah's parents decided to see a local optometrist but left feeling even more confused. "I didn't know how to relate to anything he said about Teah's vision. I didn't understand it. There I was holding a piece of paper in my hand with horrible news about my daughter's vision and visual processing ability and I didn't know what to do with it," she added.

But, instead of throwing the report away and walking away confused, Lizbeth sought the advice and second opinion of Dr. Dana Dean in San Diego.

"The night before we saw Dr. Dean was like the climax of misery for Teah," Lizbeth said. "We'd been through endless headaches, crying over homework—all the struggles."

Lizbeth describes how the night started with one little worksheet that should have taken twenty minutes. After an hour and a half, frustration had built up to a breaking point.

"Our tempers were soaring. I remember saying that it shouldn't be this hard and to just get it done, and Teah left the table and ran to her bedroom, sobbing on her bed for about fifteen minutes. She came out later and crawled into my lap. She said that I didn't understand, and I asked her to explain it to me," Lizbeth said.

Teah told her mother, "When I read it feels like there are two guns shooting me in the eyes, and then somebody sprinkles fairy dust all over me and all I want to do is go to sleep."

The next day they saw Dr. Dean. "I burst into tears in her office. They were actually tears of relief that I finally knew and understood what was wrong with Teah's vision and was happy there was something we could do to help her," Lizbeth recalled. "Vision therapy wasn't covered under our insurance plan, but how could we afford not to try it? We decided to commit to three months of vision therapy, but in only three weeks we knew things were happening," she added.

Thinking back to the first time she saw Teah, Dr. Dean described her as a "little girl lost in space." "Teah had a very low-functioning visual system overall," she said.

Teah was diagnosed with amblyopia. She had low depth perception, convergence problems, and trouble with directionality. She had double vision and was struggling with headaches.

In only eleven sessions, Teah had made great strides. Dr. Dean remembered Teah telling her at a progress evaluation that "her eyes were not making her sleepy anymore."

"We all cried," Dr. Dean added. "I cry almost every day at work. Vision therapy personally helped me and that is why I do what I do."

Dr. Dean shared that she was a straight A–student until tenth grade, when she could no longer compensate for undiagnosed vision problems. "I could not keep up with the increased workload that continued to challenge me. I could not study and remember the information even though I worked twice as hard as anyone else in my class."

"My self esteem started to go down, and I had no answers as to why this was happening. I barely scraped by during undergrad and had a very challenging time during optometry school," she recalled.

After failing her optometry board exams three times, it was suggested to her that she might have ADHD. She met with a psychiatrist who quickly prescribed medicine and cognitive therapy.

Dr. Dean shared, "It was not until I met my mentor, Dr. Robert Sanet, that I discovered my vision problem. After completing my comprehensive eye exam, he looked at me dumfounded and said, 'Dana, I don't know how you got through optometry school!' I started to cry and said to him, 'You mean to tell me that I am not stupid?'"

That was the turning point in Dr. Dean's life. She did vision therapy with Linda Sanet for nine months, and, upon taking the boards for the fourth time, she passed with flying colors!

Dr. Dean said, "Every time I meet with parents, it is my hope that they understand how much vision therapy could help their child. This was definitely true in Teah's case because she didn't have a visual system that could have led her to success."

Teah did vision therapy for almost two years. She took a three month break over one summer vacation. Teah enjoyed going to Dr. Dean's office for vision therapy, but was not a big fan of the home exercises.

Lizbeth said, "At the beginning of vision therapy, Teah had headaches, but she is such a pleaser and tried so hard to work well with her vision therapist. At first it was new and fun, but later she thought it was kind of boring because she wasn't seeing changes or results."

But, then one morning Teah suddenly realized she had not had a headache in "a really long time." She said to her mother, "Do you think vision therapy took away my headaches?" She also began to notice things while driving in the car, such as individual leaves on trees.

Dr. Dean recalled talking with Teah about the importance of the home exercises. She said, "I had to talk to her about being responsible and explain to her that *she* was the one doing the work. I told her that I was her guide." Dr. Dean believes that for anyone to be successful in vision therapy "their brain has to learn how to see it, integrate it and own it."

Though she didn't enjoy making snow angels on the floor to improve her spatial awareness, Teah continued to do all the exercises assigned by her vision therapist. She graduated from vision therapy when she was nine years old.

"She was given a book and a gift certificate, and we were all there to celebrate with her—mom, dad, sister, aunt, and both sets of grandparents," Lizbeth said.

Dr. Dean shared that Teah's final evaluation was excellent. "Her whole visual system was completely integrated. Binocular and convergence findings were within normal limits." Teah's headaches had also completely dissipated.

She had achieved 20/20-1 acuity in her left eye. "Her depth perception was measured at twenty seconds of arc, which is well within normal limits. She had convergence to the nose, which is again well within normal limits," Dr. Dean shared.

"Teah's success was so thrilling for all of us," said Lizbeth. "There are many labels that can be put on vision problems mistakenly, and it just delays the proper diagnosis. It's not just the child that suffers; it's the whole family," she added.

After vision therapy, Teah started third grade. "I had been very involved in the classroom prior to this year, but I decided to step back and let Teah step out on her own," Lizbeth said.

Teah's school had a unique report card system. Lizbeth explained, "Her report card used words like *needs refining, proficient,* and *advanced* instead of the traditional A, B, C scale. I was so excited the day her report card came home and she had earned a *proficient*. She has had no further need of *refining* since vision therapy. Third grade was a really great year!"

Jillian's Words about Teah

Our mothers say we are two peas in a pod.

We are the same age, in the same grade and we both have straight As in school. We love dogs, *Harry Potter*, and the *Twilight* series. We are both Team Jacob. Neither of us really enjoys sports that much, although Teah likes Capoeira, a Brazilian martial arts class that includes dance and music. That sounds like fun and I will check it out.

We are huge Disney fans, although growing up on opposite sides of the country, she has only been to Disneyland and I've only been to Disney World.

We both have amblyopia, and vision therapy turned our childhood nightmares into dreams of wonderful futures.

In addition to being very busy at school, Teah volunteers at the San Diego Junior Theater and has learned so much about the technical side of putting on a show. She has worked with costume, set and technical designers.

She describes herself as an avid reader, and her mom says Teah's love of reading "definitely came after vision therapy."

Lizbeth said, "I read the first chapter of *Twilight* out loud to her as I had read *Harry Potter* and other books. I was busy on work projects the few days following our first chapter of *Twilight*. I came home one evening to find her sitting in bed reading by herself. I acted like it was no big deal, but ran to tell her dad that she was reading for fun. We were practically jumping up and down. We were so excited!"

Teah loves tigers. She enjoys drawing, shopping, and even jewelry making. She told me she tries to forget her sad memories before vision therapy so she can think of all the great ones now.

To my new best friend, Teah, may your life be filled with many happy memories. Here's an idea—let's go make new memories together. I'll show you around Disney World if you'll take me to Disneyland.

To Lizbeth, you and my mom are so much alike too. Thanks for all your great advocacy efforts through the Facebook page you created, *Vision Therapy Changed My Life*. I know many people have found support and vision therapy information through your posts. And now, others can find your page as well.

Thank you for continuing to search for an answer for Teah and for reaching out to other parents with the message that vision therapy works.

Brian

"I think I was probably meant to play professional ping-pong and not hockey."

It wasn't his first big hit. As a professional hockey player for teams like the Washington Capitals, Carolina Hurricanes, Ottawa Senators, and Atlanta Thrashers, Brian had taken his share of hard hits. But on January 3, 2008, he took a hit to his face and head that changed his life.

"I was in a very vulnerable position when another player hit me with his shoulder," he said. "I actually took the hit on my cheek and my head sort of made a whiplash motion," he added.

After playing hockey for many years, he was used to injuries. This was his fourth concussion. He'd been down this road before, or so he thought. But this injury sidelined him for fifteen months and almost ended his hockey career.

"As with my other concussions, the symptoms seemed to subside over a couple of months. But when June rolled around I still felt foggy," he said. "I would feel sort of dizzy walking up stairs or pushing my kids on a swing. It was like getting off a Tilt-A-Whirl or a boat. I felt sort of seasick and my body just wasn't in a good place," he added.

Brian saw several doctors and specialists. The team trainers ultimately told him to go home for the summer and rest. "I didn't challenge myself too much. After a while, I could ride a bike, paddle a kayak. I thought I was better."

He went back to training camp that September and, after only one week, the symptoms came back. "It seemed that if I could keep my head stable, keep it still, I was okay," Brian explained. "Adding in movement was the problem."

After seeing a neurologist and finding no medical problems that could be causing his symptoms, Brian talked to Washington Capital trainer Greg Smith. "I was so frustrated and told Greg that I thought it was a problem with my eyes. I told him I could feel pressure behind my eyes," he recalled.

"Greg knew a player when they were both in Anaheim named Matt Cullen. He remembered Matt having similar problems, so Greg called him, and Matt said he had the same symptoms that I was experiencing. Matt had seen an optometrist in Raleigh named Dr. Susan Durham. So I went to see her," Brian shared.

During the evaluation with Dr. Durham, Brian sat at a computer. "She asked me what I saw on the screen," he said. "I told her nothing was crisp, so she asked me to put on a pair of glasses and look at the computer," Brian added.

"Suddenly everything was clear. I remember thinking, *Oh my gosh—this is it, this is the answer.* Everything was crisp and focused. The pressure behind my eyes went away immediately. It was like a mini-miracle!"

"She said the concussion had caused a small astigmatism and that I could wear the glasses for relief," Brian said. Dr. Durham referred him to Dr. Paul Harris in Baltimore and, in November, Brian took the weekly hour-long drive to see Dr. Harris for vision therapy.

Dr. Harris said, "Brian was moving in a guarded way, shifting his whole body from side to side to look from one point to another—something you or I would do with a quick jump of the eyes and maybe even with a small amount of head movement."

"Brian couldn't do this without getting dizzy, even with the new glasses on," Dr. Harris added. "I felt that there must be a mismatch between the signals from the balance mechanisms coming from his inner ear, the signals from his neck telling his brain where his head was on his body, and the visual signals of where the horizon was and where vertical was in his visual world."

Dr. Harris described Brian's treatment as "helping to recalibrate these three views, or where we are in space, while helping him return to the normal movement patterns with eyes moving free of his body and his head moving freely again on his torso."

"He was a great patient," Dr. Harris added.

Brian said, "I told Dr. Harris that I had a time limit. I needed to get back on the ice as soon as possible." It had already been almost a year since the concussion when Brian saw Dr. Durham, so by the time he met with Dr. Harris, time was ticking.

Dr. Harris recalled his vision therapy sessions with Brian. "Due to travel, Brian had extended sessions in the office, one-on-one with me," he said. "In each session we worked on four or five different activities designed to achieve our goals. One activity, Eye Control, had him standing with his head in a neutral position while a target was moved to extreme positions of gaze up, down, right, and left with a metronome to get him to move those eyes again."

"Brian was also asked to read off a central chart with a metronome while pointing a laser pointer to peripheral targets at a different timing pattern, using only his peripheral vision to guide the laser pointer," he added.

"In one exercise named after one of my teachers, Dr. Israel Greenwald, Brian was asked to follow a ball hanging from the ceiling that would zoom by him only inches away from his face. In one version of the activity he would have to follow the ball only with his eyes," Dr. Harris explained.

In another version of the exercise, Brian would follow the ball with his head, whipping his head side to side to keep a steady eye locked on the ball. According to Dr. Harris, this helped to reestablish Brian's ability to move his head independently of his body, which enabled him to regain routine movement patterns.

"We only did six vision therapy sessions," Dr. Harris remembers. "After two sessions, he could begin physical conditioning. After four sessions, he was cleared to begin skating and, after six sessions, he played a limited amount in rehab games with the Hershey Bears," added Dr. Harris.

Soon after starting vision therapy, Brian began hockey training in glasses, but in two or three months he didn't even need them.

Brian's first game back with the Washington Capitals was in early April. "The first couple of games back were road games," he said. "I will never forget the first home game I played after my injury. We were in the playoffs, and I scored my first goal in fifteen months. It was the game winner. My teammates were so happy for me; my coach was so proud. They put something up on the Jumbotron about it being my first goal after a fifteen-month-long injury. The crowd gave me a standing ovation. It was amazing."

After his contract with the Washington Capitals came to an end in 2010, Brian took his family to Geneva, Switzerland, where he began playing for a Swiss National League team, the Geneve-Servette.

"I was doing great and really happy to be playing hockey," he said "I'm getting older and I'd been injured, so I felt lucky to be where I was," he said.

This time the hit came on March 8, 2012, to his chin. He had his fifth concussion. "People always ask me if I could be wearing a different and better helmet or something," he said. "But I never got hit on the top of my head where the helmet would be of any help. It was to the cheek or chin."

Dr. Harris explained, "An injury on the ice is like a car accident." In many cases, hits that involve "whipping," or jerking of the head in a quick, sudden motion, are exactly like whiplash from a car accident.

"The impact of colliding with another player or hitting the boards of the rink can be compared to a low-speed traffic accident," Dr. Harris added.

Brian spent the entire month of March on his couch. "I knew while the symptoms were subsiding I needed to find an optometrist for vision therapy. I didn't know where to go in Switzerland. The doctors didn't know of anyone doing vision therapy." He told the team doctors in Geneva about his previous vision therapy success with Dr. Harris in Baltimore. "They were phenomenal doctors," Brian said. "They were very supportive and said I should follow Dr. Harris' guidance."

Dr. Harris referred Brian to an optometrist in Davos, Switzerland, which was about four and a half hours away. Flying would have been tough, possibly detrimental, so he drove to Davos. The optometrist there did a full evaluation and gave the results to Dr. Harris. After receiving the evaluation results from his colleague in Switzerland, Dr. Harris called Brian. "His instructions were to relax and heal," Brian recalls. "He told me when I got back to the states he would get me in to see an optometrist in Boston.

Brian is currently going through his second round of vision therapy with Dr. John Abbondanza.

"When I first met Brian, he told me his symptoms had gotten significantly worse after the last concussion. He had motion sickness with the slightest movement, difficulty with depth perception and complained that he was often unsure of where things were around him," said Dr. Abbondanza. "He complained of problems with walking, coordination, and balance and felt like he had to move slowly to avoid symptoms. All of these symptoms were worse with fatigue," he added.

Dr. Abbondanza recommended additional office-based optometric vision therapy, with an emphasis on visual-vestibular work and using vision to guide movement. He said, "We also wanted to work toward reducing his dependence on his eye glasses."

One of the activities involved walking on a beam wearing prism glasses—glasses that shift the world to one side. Brian's job was first to keep his balance on the beam, then to follow a swinging ball, then to keep his eyes on the swinging ball while swatting away beanbags tossed at him from both sides.

Dr. Abbondanza said that although they are still working to improve his symptoms, Brian has made tremendous gains and can now lead a more normal life.

"His situation is not unusual. Most of the patients we see with brain injury have similar symptoms of sensitivity to motion and problems with movement. The good news is that treatment is available," he added.

Jillian's Words about Brian

It is so scary to see athletes get hurt. I always flinch when I see football players knocked off their feet in a hard tackle or hockey players knocked into the walls. Brian would say that's just part of the game.

He loves hockey and he has dedicated a large part of his life to it. He keeps fighting adversity and coming back like a superhero.

Brian said, "So here I am, three and a half years after that bad concussion knocked me out of hockey, trying to recover from another injury." He describes himself as "functioning." He can do most things in moderation. Vision therapy has helped him get a little more active, but it's "baby steps this time."

"I know vision therapy works and I'm going to keep with it," Brian said.

Dr. Abbondanza said, "Brian can pretty much live his life normally now, though he may still have a way to go before he is ready to get back on the ice again competitively. One of the things that has been difficult for him is to learn to not rush the treatment. Each subsequent injury to the brain causes more numerous problems and of greater depth, and it takes longer to heal. Recovery from the first concussion is easier than from the fifth or sixth."

It may sound crazy to some people, but Brian hopes to return to Switzerland to play hockey again. I get it. Nobody wants to give up something they love. I can relate to Brian. He needs vision therapy to get back something that was lost, something that was taken from him. I needed vision therapy to give me something I'd never had. Vision therapy has changed both of our lives, just at different ages.

This time Brian sees his recovery as "getting his life back." He just wants to be healthy. He wants to run and chase his kids in the backyard. He wants to do normal, active things.

He is a strong advocate for vision therapy. He said, "I want everybody to know about vision therapy, especially athletes. It is a viable option in concussion-related injuries that isn't talked about that much." Brian adds, "Many athletes use vision therapy, not for rehab, but to correct or improve their vision and become a better player."

I always say that life is like the game Mario Kart. No matter how many times a red shell hits you, no matter how many times another character knocks you off the track, you'll always come back. Brian, I hope you will be back on the ice soon, doing what you love to do. To me you will always be a champion!

Milosz

"Hearing my son say, 'Mom, I see depth,' was one of the most exciting moments I've had in my life."
—Jennifer, Milosz's mother

You might not be impressed to hear that a sixteen-year-old boy can ride a bike and hit a baseball, but for Milosz, these accomplishments are truly astounding. Milosz has cerebral palsy and permanent brain damage from a childhood brain hemorrhage. His mother, Jennifer, an MD in family practice, said that "he has blown everyone away."

Jennifer described Milosz's birth as easy and very gentle. But when he was twelve days old, Milosz began to cry ceaselessly. "I couldn't seem to soothe him or comfort him, and I noticed that his eyes were rolling down until I could only see the whites of his eyes," she recalled.

After talking with her son's pediatrician, Jennifer rushed him to the emergency room. "His lab work was normal and he had no fever, but when they did a lumbar puncture, they kept getting blood and not spinal fluid," Jennifer shared.

An MRI showed that Milosz had a grade three massive ventricular hemorrhage. "What we were seeing with the eyes rolling back were seizures," Jennifer explained. "This type of bleeding very deep in the brain is something we see in premature babies and not full-term babies."

The news was "totally unexpected" for Jennifer and her husband, who is also a physician. Milosz was intubated, transported by ambulance to another hospital, and admitted to neonatal intensive care. "I remember that he looked so big compared to the premature babies," said Jennifer.

He stayed in intensive care for several weeks. Jennifer recalls that after he was extubated, she was able to nurse him. The fact that he would breastfeed was a good sign. A drain was put into his brain to relieve the pressure and drain the blood with the hope that he would not need a shunt (a tube that carries the cerebral spinal fluid from his brain to his stomach). Unfortunately, while in the hospital, Milosz developed a brain infection, and one step forward turned into two steps back: Milosz ended up needing a shunt.

While in the hospital, Milosz was seen by a pediatric ophthalmologist who diagnosed him with esotropia--an inward eye turn--and down-gaze paresis. At six weeks old, Milosz started patching. "It was so hard to do the patching because he would just cry and cry and cry," said Jennifer.

Upon returning home, Jennifer noticed that his eyes were rolling back or turning down again, especially when Milosz was lying down. "I called the neurosurgeon's office and they said to just have him sleep upright in his car seat. I thought that was crazy!"

Unfortunately, upon examination, doctors discovered that the fluid in his brain was draining too slowly, and Milosz needed another surgery to replace the valve for the shunt in his brain.

After Milosz's second surgery, Jennifer sought out the help of another specialist. She said, "I have a friend, Veronica, from our time in residency together, who did cranial-sacral osteopathic work with him while I held him or nursed him."

It was not long before Milosz was able to lift his head and, at age one and a half, with the help of the continuing osteopathic, occupational therapy, and physical therapy, he started to crawl and to build up his strength.

As Milosz grew older, Jennifer continued to study and research treatments that might be of help to him. She ran across the subject of vision therapy. "I had heard of vision therapy and was very curious about it. I called our ophthalmologist and he said it didn't work and to not waste our money."

But after a couple of years of physical therapy and a more holistic approach to his care, Jennifer took Milosz to see a vision therapist named Tom Headline, who worked with optometrist Dr. Bradford Murray.

"We met Tom when Milosz was three," Jennifer said. "He had an amazing gentleness, and Milosz responded so well to him."

Tom said, "I remember the first time I met Milosz. He had on little white-framed glasses and he smiled and giggled a lot." Tom said that due to Milosz's health problems, he wasn't sure exactly where to start, but he felt hopeful. "We started with the basics of learning how to aim his eyes, general movement skills, and teaching his brain how to use both eyes together."

Vision therapy is an individualized and progressive program of vision procedures. It is performed under the supervision of an optometrist and designed to fit the unique visual needs of each patient. The key word in Milosz's case is *individualized.*

"Milosz has downward gaze paresis and he had to move his whole head in order to look down. He had what I would describe as jiggly eyes that rocked back and forth."

He was diagnosed with alternating esotropia, a condition in which each eye periodically turns inward, and a vertical eye misalignment called hypertropia. Milosz's optometrist prescribed a pair of glasses with both horizontal and vertical prisms to improve his eye alignment and prescribed a program of vision therapy.

Tom said that Milosz also had weak trunk support due to his low tone cerebral palsy, so his therapy routine had to incorporate a lot of body work. Milosz had not started to walk until he was three, just prior to working with Tom. The other challenge that Milosz had was short term memory loss due to brain damage.

Jennifer explained that Milosz had brain surgery a third time. A new shunt had to be inserted into his brain, and the buildup of pressure prior to installing the new shunt resulted in even more significant brain damage.

"When he was little, I could show him blocks and he wouldn't remember anything about them a short while later," Tom said.

Time was a very difficult concept for Milosz. "I remember saying to him, 'See you next Friday,' and he would immediately turn to his mom and ask, 'Is that tomorrow?'" Tom incorporated many visual memory techniques into Milosz's vision therapy plan.

He also made the decision to do some exercises with Milosz lying flat on the ground. "When he was upright, Milosz didn't have strong trunk support, so I removed gravity from the equation by having him lie on the floor."

Tom recalled the day he noticed Milosz moving his eyes downward without moving his head. "While he was comfortably lying on the floor, I asked him to follow a ball with his eyes. I moved the ball, positioned above him, down the center line of his body and he tracked it without moving his head.

Milosz's upright body work included using a balance beam and a jump rope. "It took years for Milosz to even stand on the balance beam without falling off, but eventually he was able to do it," Tom said. "His mother and I helped him learn to jump rope. At first, I'd put the rope on the floor and his goal was to jump across it. We gradually moved up to having him jump it as we moved it. In the end, he could turn the rope and jump all by himself."

Tom believes Milosz's success in this area was a collaborative effort between his vision therapist, occupational therapist, and adaptive physical education instructor. He also gives much of the credit to Milosz.

"When his mom set her goal of doing a triathlon, Milosz discovered his own internal motivation and set a goal to run a mile," Tom said. "When he first came to vision therapy, he shuffled his feet when he walked. But now you should see him run. He is so fast!"

Tom worked with Milosz's occupational therapist to develop a coordinated approach designed to meet his needs. "It works so well when we can coordinate exercises that are helpful to the patient. I have many young patients who go to a variety of therapies each week—vision, physical, and occupational. If you add in school, homework, tutoring, and other activities, it's overwhelming. By collaborating, some of my patients can actually get most of their vision therapy home exercises done during their weekly occupational therapy appointments."

Milosz and Tom have worked together for over a decade. They still work together in the office of Dr. Benjamin Popilsky. Tom told Jennifer that he wanted to make sure Milosz still benefitted from his appointments. "Milosz was adamant in wanting to continue to work with me, and I will always be here for him," Tom said.

Jillian's Words about Milosz

Milosz is now sixteen years old, and I'm not sure I even have the words to describe my feelings about him. At first, based on his medical history, my mom and I thought Milosz used a wheelchair. Wow, were we wrong about that!

Thanks to more than a year of slow, patient help from his adaptive PE teacher, Milosz learned to ride a bike when he was eleven. He also played on a little league baseball team. When Tom heard about this, he asked Jennifer, "Can he hit the ball?" and she replied, "Absolutely!"

Although Milosz has difficulty with memory and it is very tricky for him to learn, it has not been impossible thanks to his amazing team of supporters.

I think Tom is brilliant and his work with Milosz makes me want to pursue vision therapy as a career now more than ever. Tom truly knows and understands Milosz. For example, it didn't take Tom long to realize that when doing a geo-pattern board, Milosz was building the same pattern as requested, just at a 90 degree rotation.

Tom appreciated Milosz's love of baseball, and one day stopped into a comic book store to buy baseball cards. He used them to help Milosz learn to fixate on an object.

Tom said he tells all of his young patients that it's his goal "to get you to be the boss of your eyes." Well, let me tell you what, Tom. You're the boss!

Jennifer said that one of the most exciting moments in her life was hearing Milosz say, "Mom, I see depth." I know what it means to live in a world that is no longer flat, and I am so happy he could gain fusion.

Soon after *Jillian's Story* first came out, I received an email from Jennifer about Milosz's success with vision therapy. She wrote, "We too, are a family who is HUGELY grateful for having found vision therapy." She has been an awesome mom and advocate for Milosz.

As a physician, she now understands the role vision therapy can play in changing a life and, not only does she believe in it but she also thinks it should be covered by insurance. I could hug her!

Milosz, I'm amazed by you. You run and ride bikes way better than I can. I actually failed at learning to jump rope. After getting hit in the arms and legs by that stupid rope, I couldn't seem to jump! I gave it up for my safety or maybe my sanity. I also hear you can play ping-pong.

Tom said, "We worked on eye-teaming skills for a long time. One year, while visiting family in Florida where they had a ping-pong table, Milosz was able to play."

Dude, that is amazing. You are amazing! Thank you for sharing your story.

Mary

"I didn't make eye contact with anyone for years."

Mary was in high school when she first noticed her eye drifting out.

"I noticed it while looking at myself in a mirror, and I continued to notice it every once in a while," she said.

She describes her vision as being "one eye at a time." "My brain would automatically switch between eyes. If one eye was blocked, then my other eye would take over," Mary said.

"I did find it odd that I would suddenly see things to my side that I hadn't seen even seconds before, but it had always been like that, and I thought everyone saw the way I did," she added.

Mary shared a painful memory from high school. "I had noticed this really cute boy and he came over to talk to me. As we were talking he said, 'How are you doing that with your eye?' and I wanted to die. I was so embarrassed."

Mary stopped making eye contact that day. "I just stopped looking at people. My self-esteem, my self-confidence was nonexistent," she said.

Mary's father was in the navy, and she recalled seeing the optometrist at the base when she was in junior high. "He prescribed glasses with a lens that was so thick just on one side that it made my left eye look giant compared to my right one. I hated wearing them and I was so self-conscious."

Mary said she wasn't very social in school, but that she did not do too poorly academically. "I had a tendency to daydream quite a bit," she admitted. She remembers feeling frustrated that her brother barely studied while she did hours of homework every night. "My brother hardly had to try and he made better grades than me," she shared.

"When I graduated from high school I had absolutely no interest in going to college. I got a job as a cashier at a grocery store," she said. Then someone suggested she apply for an open position as a lab tech in water and wastewater with the local utility company. He mentioned it every time he saw me for several weeks, but I kept thinking they wouldn't hire someone without experience," she said.

She finally gave in to his suggestion and applied for the job. "The company waited for three months to fill the position, but I was the only one who ever applied, so they offered me the job and trained me. I feel so lucky and blessed to have fallen into this career," Mary said.

"I remember having trouble out in the field whenever we needed to drain water from a tank. The instructions were to drain the tank by two feet and, if there weren't markings on the tank, I couldn't figure out how to do it," she said. Her coworkers offered her tips and suggestions on how to judge the measurement, but she couldn't visualize it.

"A friend of mine told me years ago about vision therapy, but when I searched for information about it, I couldn't find anything," she said.

When Mary was about twenty-one years old, she saw an optometrist, who told her she was using one eye at a time.

"He said it, but then moved on to talk about other things. He didn't say I had amblyopia, and he didn't tell me about vision therapy," Mary said.

A few years later, she had Lasik surgery, which she said helped her some, but she continued to wonder about vision therapy.

Mary said she continued to struggle with making eye contact. "When I met the man who would be my husband, we talked for hours the first night we met," she said. "After we had been dating for three months, he asked me to marry him."

"I said yes, of course, but I also felt obligated to talk to him about my wandering eye. I sat him down on the couch and told him there was something he might not have noticed about me, but that I needed to tell him. It was so awkward and I struggled to tell him about my eye. He said, "Oh, that's no big deal. I've noticed that."

Mary and her husband have laughed about that moment for years. "He said he didn't know where I was going with that confession, but my eye didn't bother him at all," she giggled.

About ten years after searching for vision therapy information the first time, Mary tried again. "This time I found some websites about vision therapy that led me to Dr. James Horning," she shared.

Dr. Horning said, "Mary first came to my office when she was thirty-seven years old. She was concerned that her left eye was drifting out more, especially when she was tired. Mary had a condition called anisometropia, where one eye was much more farsighted than the other eye. This usually results in amblyopia, or lazy eye. The vision in one eye doesn't develop as well as the other eye. The brain will also turn off or ignore the input from the amblyopic eye. In most cases the eyes will remain straight. Mary's case was different because not only did her brain ignore or suppress the input from her left eye, her eye turned way up and out."

"Mary's main goal for considering vision therapy was to give her the ability to keep her eyes straight. What I didn't know at the time was that she secretly wanted to be able to see 3D movies and experience the depth. One very exciting point in the vision therapy process was the time Mary had spent the weekend at Universal Studios and was able to see the images popping out of the movie screen. She was so excited when she described the experience to our staff," Dr. Horning added.

"There was a time in my career when I would have been apprehensive about the chance of success with a case like Mary's because she had the condition for a very long time. What I have found is that age is not a limiting factor in treating strabismus or amblyopia. I think the cognitive level of the patient plays a big part in treatment. Adults can be more successful than young children because they are more motivated and they have a higher level of understanding when it comes to the vision therapy procedures. They understand how to perform the procedures correctly and what they are looking for when they do the procedures, so they're better able to figure out what they need to do to be successful at a vision therapy exercise," he said.

"Mary experienced many positive benefits from vision therapy in addition to straight eyes and depth perception. Her reading has improved in that she loses her place less frequently, her oral reading is smoother, and she isn't as tired when she reads. She also notices less letter reversal and is more comfortable driving. All of these gains have given her more self-confidence and self-esteem," he added.

Mary said, "Dr. Horning said we could be successful if we could train my brain to make my eyes work together. I had no stereo vision and couldn't see 3D."

Dr. Horning said Mary was successful with vision therapy because she worked very hard. He said, "Either in our office or at home or even in her work place she was able to do the exercises every day. The consistency really paid off."

"There were many vision therapy procedures that Mary responded to well. One that we have success with in these types of cases is "projected vectograms." In this procedure, Mary was placed in a dark room where two similar images were projected on a large screen at one end of the room. Special polarized glasses are worn that allow the right eye to see one image and the left eye to see the other image. The images are so big that it is almost impossible for the brain to ignore the input from the lazy eye," he described.

"The images were then moved so they corresponded to the exact orientation of Mary's eyes. This allowed the brain to put together the image from one eye with the image from the other eye. This is usually the first time that the brain is looking at the same image out of each eye at the same time. With repeated exposures, the image will begin to move out of the wall and appear to float in the middle of the room, like images in a 3D movie. For someone like Mary who has not seen depth before, it is a very powerful experience. Needless to say Mary really enjoyed this procedure," he added.

"I am so glad I found Dr. Horning and I hope vision therapy becomes more mainstream," Mary said.

Jillian's Words about Mary

Dr. Horning was my optometrist too! Mary was in great hands.

Mary didn't find vision therapy until she was in her mid-thirties, but it proved to be very successful for her. She can use both of her eyes together now and can see 3D. Stereo vision really makes a difference in how we see.

"The best part is driving," Mary said. "Now when I approach a red light, I can judge where to stop even if nobody is in front of me," she added. She used to stop way early and drift forward toward cars in front of her or toward the traffic light.

She liked to take one of her vision therapy exercises to work. It is a transparency of a thick rope curled up in a circle. She would find it frustrating that her coworkers could see the 3D effect right away, but eventually she got it. It actually became really easy for her. She gets the really cool effect with the rope exercise of seeing the rope jump out closer to her—about halfway toward her body.

She looks forward to going back to one of her favorite places, Universal Orlando, and watching the 3D movies.

Dr. Horning said, "Mary continues to wear glasses that have prism in the lenses. The prism lenses make it easier for Mary to keep her eyes straight. The exciting thing is that Mary can take off her glasses and keep her eyes straight without them. Before therapy, Mary's left eye would always point up and out. Over time we will continue to reduce the amount of prism in her glasses."

Mary is thrilled that her eye no longer wanders unless she is extremely tired. She is happy that she "looks normal" and it's done wonders for her self-esteem. She went to college and graduated with all As except for one B. She continues to move ahead in her career, and I am so happy for her.

Mary should have been referred to vision therapy years ago. She should never have made it through vision screenings, but screenings are not good enough.

Dr. David A. Damari, President of the College of Optometrists in Vision Development (COVD) said, "We are well into the twenty-first century, yet we are still using a benchmark from the 1800s to determine if a child can see well enough to learn. Standing twenty feet from an eye chart is not enough to adequately test children's vision."

COVD reminded parents during their National Vision and Learning Month campaign that "many children can pass school vision screenings or vision screenings at the pediatrician's office but still have one or more of a variety of vision disorders that impact how their two eyes work together when they read. This is because vision screenings are not designed to test all seventeen visual skills that are necessary for success in school. Typically vision screenings only test for visual acuity (how clearly letters can be seen from a distance of twenty feet away), which is only one of these seventeen visual skills."

Mary was also let down by the two optometrists she saw prior to Dr. Horning. I think all optometrists need to get on the same page when it comes to vision therapy. My mom told someone the other day that, although we chose to write about twenty-two people in our book, we could have written about twenty-two thousand. Vision therapy is working and people are achieving amazing, life-changing results. I think all optometrists have an obligation to know what their peers are doing in this field. To me, there are eye doctors and then there are eye doctors who are vision and brain experts.

To Mary, thank you for sharing your story. I'm glad the third time was the charm when it came to finding the right optometrist. Universal Orlando is one of my favorite places on earth, and I'd love to meet you there someday for some 3D movies and roller coasters.

Noah

"I was worried I would have double vision for the rest of my life."

He had an MRI the day before he left for college and moved into his dorm room without knowing the results.

"When I was eighteen, I suddenly started having double vision," said Noah. "I had been wearing glasses since the end of kindergarten, so when I went to see an ophthalmologist, he just made my lenses stronger," he added.

When that ophthalmologist learned that the new lenses were making things even worse, he sent Noah to see another ophthalmologist. Noah recalled, "The second doctor sent me for an MRI just to be safe. I used to do a lot of short track speed skating and, when I suddenly started having double vision, I wondered if I'd hit my head harder than I realized at some point. My parents and I had a theory that my double vision could be the result of a head injury from skating."

But, as the MRI would show, their theory was incorrect. Luckily, Noah did not have a brain injury. He was sent back for another appointment with the same ophthalmologist who had changed his lenses and this time the doctor's recommendation was surgery.

"He said I had strabismus, an eye turn," said Noah. "My mother and I talked recently about my childhood. She said that I got glasses after my first trip to an optometrist at age six. My parents took me to the eye doctor because I had recently started getting headaches and they noticed that I would hold things very close when reading and writing," he added.

Noah was told to use his glasses just for close work. "Evidently, I didn't like wearing them because I had to take them off to see the blackboard. A year or so later they put me in bifocals, which I was better about wearing," Noah shared.

Noah recalls having trouble learning to read when he was young, but overall he did well in school. He graduated high school and went on to college.

"We put off the recommended surgery because I was just starting college," Noah said. Even with double vision he was doing well in his classes. His vision problem was worse at a distance, so he could read fairly well.

"I had to sit super close to the board," Noah recalls of those days. "I tilted my head at an angle to see. Any information I couldn't see I got from friends later. They knew I had a funky vision problem because of my really thick glasses and they'd helped me with notes."

Noah had "lots of headaches." Because he'd endured frequent headaches since the age of five, he did not think much about them. It was just the way it was. "I remember the first year of college as such an odd experience."

One day, Noah called an optometrist close to campus to get his glasses fixed. "He said eighteen diopters of prism in my lenses was crazy!" Noah said. "We talked about vision therapy and he sent me to see a behavioral optometrist, Dr. Theresa Ruggiero. He said that if I have double vision I should go to Dr. Ruggiero because she has helped lots of people with vision problems through vision therapy." Noah saw Dr. Ruggiero for the first time in January of his freshman year.

"I was there for several hours," he recalls. "Dr. Ruggiero took the time to really explain everything and we talked about the best plan for me." At first they discussed doing vision therapy twice a week, but Noah felt that schedule would really interfere with school. They agreed on a plan that included vision therapy sessions once a week and fifteen to twenty minutes of "homework" almost every day.

"I remember friends coming by my dorm room to try out some of my exercises," said Noah. "I had exercises that involved using a ball on a string. It was supposed to be hung over my head, but I had nowhere in the dorm room to hang it," he added. "I would always find a friend to hold it up in the air for me."

In addition to helping him with vision therapy exercises, his friends would drive him to vision therapy once a week. "It was tough because Dr. Ruggiero's office was too far away to walk and I had to get rides. I couldn't drive with double vision," explained Noah.

Driving was never comfortable for him. "Even before I had double vision, we all had doubts about this for me. I was a very hesitant driver (I was very hesitant with lots of things) and my parents practically had to force me to practice driving. I think a large part of it was that I had difficulty with spatial relationships in general. Add in figuring out where things are in relation to your car, which is large and moving fast."

Eventually Noah overcame his hesitation in many departments and gained an incredible amount of confidence. "Luckily, I had a community of people helping me when I didn't drive," he added.

One member of Noah's wonderful support system was Dr. Sue Barry. "Dr. Sue," as she is widely known today, is the author of *Fixing My Gaze: A Scientist's Journey into Seeing in Three Dimensions*.

Noah recalled, "Dr. Barry taught at my college. She was on a sabbatical and offered to drive me to vision therapy. She was writing her book at the time, and she'd work on it while I was in my appointments." Later in Noah's collegiate career, Dr. Sue became his academic adviser.

"Sue also provided quite a bit of emotional support when I was going through vision therapy, and we would meet periodically and discuss vision and how vision therapy works, which also sparked my interest in neuroscience as a major and vision therapy as a career," Noah said.

According to Dr. Barry, she met Noah when he was a first-year student. "Our optometrist, Theresa Ruggiero, mentioned that she was taking on a new patient and asked if I would talk to him and his parents. When we spoke, I offered to drive Noah back and forth to vision therapy. Why did I offer to drive? Because vision therapy can transform a person's life," she added. Dr. Sue is currently driving another student to vision therapy and the sessions are helping this student too.

Thinking back to his early days in vision therapy, Noah said, "After about two months, I noticed my headaches were less. Early on in vision therapy, I had moments without double vision and I felt so hopeful that it would work. It was a huge relief because I was worried that I'd have double vision for the rest of my life."

After doing vision therapy for the rest of that semester, he went home for the summer. Back in the Boston area, Noah did a few months of vision therapy with Dr. Cathy Stern before returning to college.

"I continued through my whole sophomore year without a break and took time off my junior year. I had reached a point where I really wasn't the most dedicated vision therapy patient." Noah said. "I wasn't where I wanted to end up, but I could see most of the time without double vision. I still wasn't driving, but I was doing better. In most situations, my double vision and my headaches were a lot better," Noah remembered.

Noah enrolled for three more months of vision therapy during the spring semester of his junior year. He said, "When I finished vision therapy, they left me with some maintenance therapy to do occasionally, especially if I began having more symptoms. They assumed that I wouldn't regress totally, but they left me with a few things in case I needed a "tune-up."

By this time, Noah had developed a strong interest in optometry and his vision was at its best.

"At first I wondered if my interest in optometry was more academic and I thought about using my degree for research, but after college I started working for Dr. Cathy Stern. She trained me to be a vision therapist."

Dr. Stern said, "Noah was a very dedicated patient, and I watched how vision therapy made him more confident in his daily life. Without hesitation, I later hired him as a vision therapist, and he made every patient feel special and secure. He's now in optometry school, and I know he will be a very skilled and compassionate doctor."

Jillian's Words about Noah

Good for Noah! How many college students would look for an answer to their vision issues like he did? I like picturing all of his college friends helping him with vision therapy exercises.

I did the ball-on-a-string exercises in my vision therapy homework sessions just like Noah. My parents worried that the kitchen light fixture would come crashing down whenever I hung the ball from it. It never did. I remember one time that my mom stood on a chair and held the ball in the air for me, but that didn't work as well as having it swing from the chandelier.

I'm glad Noah had lots of friends to help him, including Dr. Sue. Having Dr. Sue Barry drive you to vision therapy is like having Harry Potter take you to wizard lessons!

Now Noah drives himself wherever he wants to go. He enjoys movies, concerts, and plays, which he once found "horrible and distracting."

The other really cool thing about Noah is that he is now a second year optometry student at the New England College of Optometry.

About being a vision therapist, he said, "It was so much fun, a really great career. Vision therapy is challenging, rewarding, and engaging," Noah said. It's not that Noah didn't love being a vision therapist; he just found that he wanted to pursue it as a Doctor of Optometry.

Noah said, "It was actually a very tough decision to leave vision therapy to go to optometry school. I had wonderful experiences as a vision therapist and it was very hard to leave that. But I really wanted to learn more about optometry and vision and other ways to help people."

When asked what she thought about Noah's choice to attend optometry school, Dr. Sue said, "I think it's great that Noah is in optometry school. He's whip smart and a hard worker. Combine those qualities with his own experiences with vision therapy and he will make an outstanding optometrist. I'm very proud of him!"

Vision therapy is a big part of my life and I think I would like to be an optometrist someday. This is a really hard goal for me because I will have to study human anatomy on cadavers and I think that's sort of creepy. I didn't even know what the word "cadaver" meant until I took my first optometry college tour at Northeastern State University College of Optometry in Oklahoma. I didn't realize doctors study and learn in such a way. But it makes sense. Optometry students have told me not to worry about that for now and not to let my fear get in the way of my goals. I'm really grateful to learn from several students that "if they can do it, so can I."

Noah would tell you straight up that vision therapy changed his life. "Vision is your world in a lot of ways and it's true that when you are insecure in your vision you are insecure in everything else. The world just seemed a lot more daunting. I cannot imagine what my life would be like now if vision therapy had not been part of it. I can honestly say I am a different person now, and so, so, so much better off—happier, balanced, at peace—for it!"

I really admire Noah for changing direction in his career so that he can learn more and do more for others. When I asked him for advice, he told me to work very hard in school and ask lots of questions. So here is a question: what is the definition of *hero*? It is a person admired for brave or helpful deeds, a person with noble qualities. That makes you a hero, Noah, and I know you'll change many, many lives just like ours!

R. J.

"Nobody could find him at school. He was hiding in a closet."
—Betty, R. J.'s mother

Today, R. J. is a happy nine-year-old boy. Unfortunately, "happy" is not a word his family would have picked to describe him two years ago.

When R. J. was little, he went to kindergarten like most children. But he found very little to like about it.

"His teacher couldn't figure him out," his mother, Betty, remembers. "He had many learning inconsistencies, and we wondered if it was a language issue. We spoke Spanish to him at home and English wasn't his first language."

R. J. wasn't just struggling to learn, he was troubled and having meltdowns at school. He often hid under his desk or under tables. "He tried everything to avoid schoolwork," Betty recalls. "One day his reading tutor came to work with him and nobody could find him. He was hiding in a closet," she added.

"We took him to a doctor for an evaluation, and we were told he had receptive-expressive disorder," Betty shared.

Simply put, children with receptive-expressive disorder have trouble expressing their thoughts and understanding messages from others.

"R. J. went for a neuropsych evaluation, and that doctor agreed with the receptive-expressive disorder diagnosis and added in Attention Deficit Disorder (ADD)," Betty recalled. At that point, R. J. started speech therapy and a reading program. Betty recalled that the psychologist gave R. J. some coping skills to use at school, such as "using his words" to express himself.

"I went to a parent-teacher conference in March of his first grade year, and his teacher said that R. J. wasn't learning anything," Betty said. "I was so angry to find this out in March, so far into the school year, and to discover they weren't using any of the skills or tools he needed," she added.

R. J. began second grade in a different school. Two weeks into classes, his teacher said that he was not ready for second grade. The school's recommendation was to have him repeat first grade.

"We didn't want to put him back in first grade. I was worried that R. J. would feel horrible about being held back," Betty said. "I didn't want a sense of failure to be stuck with him," she added.

But while visiting R. J.'s classroom on open house night, Betty discovered something shocking. "I sat at his desk and noticed all of his pencils were chewed up and his papers were all wadded into balls," she shared. "I was so upset and worried about him and I left the classroom in tears. We made the decision to move him back to first grade," Betty said.

The decision to have R. J. repeat first grade proved to be a good one. The best part of this year came in the form of a reading specialist named Peggy. A former special ed teacher trained in dyslexia, Peggy began working with R. J.

"R. J. is a very bright kid, just a little quirky," said Peggy. "He had such trouble reading, such anxiety. It was a laborious task for him," she added.

Peggy recalls how R. J. would push away books and physically turn away from her. "His eyes would take on an almost frightful look. He had a complete repulsion toward books," she added.

She noticed that R. J.'s tracking was impaired. "He had no fluency when he read," Peggy said. "He had to sound out every word, even if that word was repeated a number of times in the same passage."

One day Peggy asked R. J. if any of the words were floating on the page. He looked at her in surprise. "I had a feeling that something was wrong with R. J.'s vision," she said. "My daughter had struggled to read when she was little and we took her to vision therapy to treat convergence insufficiency. My brother and sister were both in vision therapy when they were young. I know it works," she said.

Peggy recommended to R. J.'s parents that he have a comprehensive eye exam.

R. J. first saw Dr. Neil Margolis in September 2011. "Dr. Margolis diagnosed R. J. with amblyopia and explained to us why R. J. couldn't read, why 3D movies bothered him," Betty recalled.

Dr. Margolis said, "I received a note from R. J.'s reading tutor explaining that it seemed R. J. had to fight to keep his eyes on the page. He could only look at the page for a short time and then had to look away. R. J. presented as a bright boy who lacked confidence. He had to be redirected to task and was creative."

R. J. had been treated for amblyopia when he was very young by an ophthalmologist who suggested patching. R. J. wore a patch over his stronger eye to force the weaker one to work.

Dr. Margolis said, "From a visual standpoint what struck me about R. J. was the fact that there was strong suppression of his right eye on all binocular vision tests despite his years of patching."

Dr. Margolis diagnosed R. J. with refractive amblyopia, suppression of binocular vision, and oculomotor dysfunction.

R. J. began vision therapy in October 2011, and his latest formal progress evaluation was in January 2013. The evaluation revealed that his visual acuity had improved in his amblyopic eye and his binocular vision no longer showed any suppression. He was using both eyes as he should.

After the first few weeks in vision therapy, R. J. began to find school a little easier. "It was easier for him to copy from the board, and his frustration level went way down," Betty said.

When R. J. started second grade, he was assigned to the same teacher who had recommended he repeat first grade. "R. J. was worried that she would send him back to first grade again, but that didn't happen." This time, second grade was a much better year for R. J.

R. J.'s parents wish they had known about developmental optometry and had started R. J. in vision therapy from the very beginning of his struggles. Betty said, "Even when Peggy told us about vision therapy, R. J.'s ophthalmologist said we should not do vision therapy. She said the only thing that works is patching and eye drops."

"He is a different child now," Betty said. "I was surprised to see the improvement in his visual-perceptual scores from a year ago. He is reading and so grateful to his vision therapist, Anne," she added.

R. J. continues to work with his tutor, Peggy. She has seen a tremendous change in him thanks to vision therapy.

"I'm a teacher and I have personally seen vision therapy make amazing differences in a child's ability to learn," Peggy said. "In R. J.'s case, as in many cases, vision therapy removed an obstacle preventing him from learning. R. J. still has other learning challenges, but having his vision corrected will help remediate the other areas." R. J.'s current diagnosis is ADD with a reading and writing disorder, but he is no longer considered to have receptive-expressive disorder.

"It's imperative that we reach teachers, parents, and doctors about vision therapy. Screenings are inadequate and, as a rule, pediatricians are not advocates of vision therapy. That has got to change," Peggy added.

Jillian's Words about R. J.

R. J. is now nine years old and according to his mom, he is doing "amazing."

I have amblyopia like R. J. and I also wore a patch when I was young. I was patched eleven hours every day for three years, from age six through age nine. R. J. had so many vision problems similar to mine. He was developmentally delayed because of his vision.

Dr. Margolis explains, "The basic foundation for visual-spatial referencing, understanding right and left sides of his body, and how to project this concept into his surroundings was clearly delayed."

R. J. and children with similar vision problems often have trouble in school. They struggle with tracking, judging how many words will fit on a line or how much space to leave between words, and finding their place while copying from the board.

Other learning difficulties might include losing your place when reading; reversing letters, words, and numbers; holding reading material close to your face; and skipping and repeating words.

In his recent follow-up evaluation, R. J. was able to track a very challenging pattern of numbers and still keep his place. He couldn't do it prior to vision therapy.

Dr. Margolis said that R. J. is now more self-assured, more confident in his responses, and more willing to engage in visual tasks. He is also more willing to take on challenging tasks.

"I am proud of him for the changes he has achieved through hard work, and his mother should be commended for her diligence," said Dr. Margolis.

I am so happy for R. J. It really broke my heart to learn that he used to hide at school. In fourth grade, I went to the restroom everyday to basically hide or get away from math class. I completely understand the frustration, anxiety, and fear R. J. used to have.

We are so much alike. Not only do we share childhood vision struggles, but we have seen our struggles lessened or erased thanks to vision therapy. We both love animals, Disney World, roller-coasters (except R. J. doesn't like the ones that go upside down), and the TV show *MythBusters.*

Like me, R. J. now loves school. Maybe love is too strong a word for how any kid feels about school, but he likes it.

R. J. said, "I didn't always like school. It used to be really hard for me. Reading made it really hard and I would get confused and stuck."

He especially likes social studies. His teachers, Mrs. Lencioni, Mrs. B, and Mrs. Henry, have helped him so much and he is really grateful to them. He is developing into a reader and told me he liked *Sports Illustrated Kids 3D Sports Blast,* which I thought must be a boy thing because I had never heard of it. I looked it up and there are some cool 3D pictures of athletes.

Though R. J. and I were young when vision therapy came into our lives, we weren't too young to realize and appreciate what a difference it made. We are both thankful to our doctors and vision therapists and, most of all, to our parents. Without them, we would not have done vision therapy at all.

To R. J., I want to say that nothing can stop you now, and the life you have ahead of you will be wonderful! No more hiding—it's time to fly!

Whitney

"My eyes look straight and have since I was three."

Whitney had strabismus surgery when she was three years old to correct an eye turn. "They thought it was a success because my eyes looked straight," she said.

Whitney's parents, Dawn and Brad, said their daughter was never a fussy baby; she seemed quite content just to sit and watch everything going on around her. Although she crawled as expected, she didn't start walking until she was eighteen months old.

"Some friends of ours called her Spud because she was a couch potato when she was little," Brad said.

As she got older, Whitney tried many sports such as volleyball and soccer, but she wasn't the best of players. "She wanted to be on the team but wasn't the go-getter. She wasn't an aggressive player at all, although she went to all the practices and became frustrated when she was not played," Brad said.

Whitney recalled numerous struggles in school. "My grades weren't great even though I really tried," she said. "Nobody could ever figure out my learning problems." Whitney saw an optometrist when she was in fourth grade and he prescribed glasses, but she didn't like wearing them. The optometrist did not mention vision therapy to Whitney and her parents.

Describing Whitney as a very intelligent and verbally bright child, Dawn said, "We thought her school problems and the fact that she scored below average on tests were because she is an auditory learner," Dawn recalled.

One day during middle school, one of Whitney's teachers set up a game of Jeopardy for the class. "She answered the most difficult questions of the day that other students in previous classes had not been able to answer," said Brad. "We thought it was her learning style— auditory. When the teacher asked her how she knew the answer, she replied, 'I heard it on the news.' We never once thought it could be a vision problem."

Whitney recalled having extreme difficulties with math as she got into middle school and high school. "I was doing okay in math and then we moved from Bend to Salem, Oregon. My new school had math class every day instead of every other day and I was completely lost."

She struggled in English because reading and writing were difficult for her, and she had to work very hard to learn those skills. "Reading was a problem for me because if I read for too long I'd either get a headache or I'd get sleepy and fall asleep," Whitney shared. "I only read what I had to for class. I never read for fun."

"We thought she might have ADD, but testing showed she did not. They said she had a comprehension problem," Dawn said.

High school became so difficult for Whitney that she wanted to give up. Her parents recalled the day she told them, "I'm done with school."

"We were so worried about her and immediately called her counselor at school. He was extremely helpful, suggesting things that would keep her going in school and motivate her in the right direction. He rearranged her schedule and helped her stay in school and on track," Dawn said.

Brad describes Whitney's driver's education as a "very traumatic experience."

"She couldn't pass the written test to get her permit. I think she tried three times. Then the man at the DMV told her they had an audio version of the test and that she could take it. She made a 95!"

But Whitney never liked driving. Actually, she hated it. Brad said, "I took her out for test drives that only ended in failure. Then she was enrolled in private driving lessons. When it was time to take her driving test, she never left the parking lot.

"We dropped her off for her test and came back an hour later. She was sitting in the car in the same parking spot with the woman from DMV. She rolled down her window, and I asked how Whitney had done. She said, 'We never moved the car.'"

Despite her struggles, Whitney graduated from high school. She went to college but quit after a year because it wasn't for her. "After that, I went to beauty school, but I never got my license because I had such a hard time passing the state tests," she shared.

In her early twenties, she saw a specialist in Portland about her learning difficulties and he sent her to an optometrist, who said she needed vision therapy.

"I didn't do anything about it at the time because I was moving to Bend," said Whitney. She got a job at a health club, and one of her friends there mentioned that he was in vision therapy with Dr. Gabby Marshall. Whitney made an appointment to see her.

"I remember sitting in the waiting room at Dr. Marshall's office and there was a poster on the wall about *Jillian's Story* and I wanted to read it," she said.

Dr. Marshall said that Whitney presented with an intermittent esotropia. She said, "I've seen patients like her with this type of inconsistency, and we've had much success with vision therapy."

"The problem with strabismus surgery is that patients and their parents have the impression that once they've had surgery, they are fixed and good to go. But, visually, it's not about what they can surgically do to the muscles; it's what you can do with the brain," Dr. Marshall explained.

Dr. Marshall does not believe strabismus surgery is necessary. "Vision therapy is nonsurgical, noninvasive, and has little risk," she said. "There is always a risk when you go under general anesthesia, and some claim there could be a link between repeated anesthesia and learning disabilities in children. Sixty percent of children from infants to the age of five will outgrow their esotropia and if they don't, strabismus is treatable without surgery. It happens every day!"

Whitney enrolled in vision therapy and went twice a week. Her vision therapist, Erin, recalled that Whitney wanted to improve her processing speed at work. "Whitney shared with me that she didn't seem to catch on as quickly as she wished, so we also worked on a process of fixate, solve, and express," she said.

"Whitney lacked confidence at times, and I had to convince her that it was okay to be wrong. We worked hard with small trampolines, balance boards, and circle of concentration activities too," said Erin.

During vision therapy, Whitney read Dr. Sue Barry's book *Fixing My Gaze* and found she could relate to Sue. "I read the part in her book about seeing the snow falling and seeing individual leaves on trees and I looked around and thought I was seeing it right. But then one day, as I was driving home from vision therapy, I thought, *Wow, I wasn't seeing things right.*

Whitney graduated from vision therapy after only six months, with her parents there to celebrate with her. Erin said, "Whitney has changed. Not only visually, but she is so much more engaging." Her parents agree.

"As we left Dr. Marshall's office after her vision therapy graduation, she was leading the way. She has become a dynamic, outgoing and confident young woman. We are so proud of her," said Dawn.

Jillian's Words about Whitney

I am so glad Whitney wrote to me. She is so sweet and supportive of my goal of spreading the news about vision therapy. She is now twenty-six years old. She said she was such a stubborn child that it's probably better that she did vision therapy as an adult, but her parents think it would have been immensely helpful to have known about her vision problems earlier in life.

"When Whitney gave us your book, *Jillian's Story*, we read it and were stunned at how much it fit Whitney. It was the missing link," said Brad.

"Whitney has struggled with learning all her life, and I don't think she has ever thought about all of the options available to her," Brad shared. He and Dawn are thrilled that she can now successfully pursue anything she wants.

"I haven't decided what I want to study, but I think I'd like to give college another try," Whitney said.

She is doing really well now. She is a confident driver, learns faster at her job, and doesn't get headaches while reading. Her depth perception and peripheral vision have dramatically improved.

Whitney recalled going to a 3D movie a few years ago, prior to vision therapy. "I wondered what everyone was talking about," she said. Now she knows.

I can't imagine going all the way through my childhood with undiagnosed vision problems. I've talked to many young adults who say they had poor self-esteem and few career choices. That's sad. I hope we can tell enough people of all ages, especially parents, teachers, and guidance counselors, that anyone struggling in school should have a comprehensive eye exam with an optometrist.

I am a huge advocate for early childhood comprehensive eye exams and I think all kids should see an optometrist before they start school. Very few states require eye exams before kids start school.

Until 2012, Missouri had a law requiring children to see an eye doctor of their choice prior to starting kindergarten. The law was strongly opposed by pediatricians, ophthalmologists, and some school nurses. They said a vision screening was adequate, but I am living proof that it is not.

I had four vision screenings when I was four and five years old—two at my preschool and two at my pediatrician's office—and nobody caught the fact that I had amblyopia. They either said I was fine or claimed I was not very cooperative.

My mom went to Missouri to testify in favor of their state law, and she was really disturbed and upset to see all the doctors in their white lab coats lobbying at the capitol against required eye exams for children.

The law no longer exists. Someone tried to explain it to me by saying that it wasn't fair to parents to require that they pay for an eye exam for their child. I'm sure it was more complicated than that because laws require parents to take their kids for immunizations prior to school and student athletes have to get physicals before they can play sports.

How did everything get so messed up? There should be no more political fights. A child's job is to learn and they can't do that when they can't see correctly. Doctors should do what is best for kids, not what seems adequate, and parents must demand that they do so.

Whitney's dad, Brad, said, "There is no reason not to pursue vision therapy if your child is struggling. Give it a chance."

He believes that schools should give comprehensive eye exams priority over tests for learning problems. He is right. Many vision problems are misdiagnosed as learning problems. You can't fix a visual learning problem at school, no matter how good the teacher or tutor may be.

To Whitney, I say that the world is yours now. Stay confident and dream new dreams. I think they will come true.

Marc

"I was the kid who couldn't seem to pay attention."

In first grade, teachers constantly told Marc to sit still, stop humming, and stop whistling. They accused him of lapses in attention; his behavior was becoming a problem. They told his mother that he was "either an idiot or that he had problems" and suggested that he take a vision test.

"School was tough," Marc said. "Reading was especially hard." Teachers told Marc's mother, Eilene, that he had trouble with phonics and would need to learn to sight-read. In second grade, they said he was good with verbal instructions but not written ones.

Marc's mother took these not-so-kind words to heart and took her son to see an optometrist. The optometrist knew something was amiss with Marc's focusing and eye teaming, so he sent Marc to Dr. Eliot Forest, an expert in New York. Dr. Forest identified at least three vision issues including an ocular motor problem, accommodative insufficiency, and difficulty with laterality and directionality, all of which were treatable with vision therapy.

"I remember my first doctor, Dr. Forest, and traveling after school, fighting New York traffic to get there," said Marc. He recalls Dr. Forest's office was not big, but the waiting room was always packed with kids and parents.

When Dr. Forest passed away suddenly, Marc was forced to change vision therapy providers. Dr. Joel Waldstreicher of Long Island, NY, "picked up right where Dr. Forest had left off."

Marc said he remembers all the vision therapy equipment in Dr. Waldstreicher's office. "I was like a tornado! I would touch everything and wanted to know what each piece of equipment would do. I remember vectograms, but most of all I remember that he had a prism reader. It's an old-time projector with a film strip. I would watch and read and answer comprehension questions later."

"I did vision therapy on one of the original orthoptic programs," Marc said. "The equipment in his office was awesome."

Eilene describes Dr. Waldstreicher's office in a different way. "If you walked into his office, you'd think a bomb had just gone off. But the man was a genius," she added.

Marc wore bifocals from second grade through high school. At eighteen, he started wearing progressive lenses. "I still wear progressive lenses. I don't need them to see. In other words, I don't need them for my acuity. I need them for my visual processing. I can focus for longer periods of time and not get a headache if I wear them," he added.

Marc saw Dr. Waldstreicher off and on throughout his years in school, and the visits made a tremendous difference in his ability to progress and succeed. "In elementary school, I had trouble reading and couldn't even read my own handwriting, but I did vision therapy and kept moving ahead," Marc said.

His mother recalls that, up until fourth grade, the school didn't seem to expect much of Marc. Eileen said, "At the beginning of fourth grade, his teacher called me in on the second day of school. She was a throwback, old-school teacher that was not going to let Marc slide by. She told me it was going to be a tough year for us because she was going to make Marc work hard."

Thanks to that fourth grade teacher and vision therapy sessions with Dr. Waldstreicher, Marc went from falling behind in school to getting ahead. Eilene recalls, "School was one challenge after another, and I don't know what we would have done without Dr. Waldstreicher and vision therapy. He always had ideas to help Marc be successful. He was the only kid in school that was allowed to use an Apple computer in class," she added.

Dr. Waldstreicher recommended the Apple computer to help Marc take notes and learn without the constraints of his handwriting. He also asked the school to let Marc use a ruler on bubble tests and other projects where his vision was an issue.

Marc truly began to soar in middle and high school. He continued to see Dr. Waldstreicher from time to time.

"When he was in high school he wanted to take an honors course, but the school said no to him," Eilene recalled. "I asked them what was the worst thing that could happen and suggested they let him try. He did great!"

Marc graduated high school and was accepted to Washington University in St. Louis. He went to college as a pre-med major but decided within a few months that he didn't want to be a medical doctor. He wanted to be an optometrist.

"Vision therapy opened the door for me to succeed in middle school, high school, college and beyond," said Marc. "I think about the fact that now, as an optometrist, I am helping others like Dr. Waldstreicher helped me. I think about it every day!"

Dr. Marc Taub is an associate professor and Chief of the Vision Therapy and Rehabilitation Service at The Eye Center at the Southern College of Optometry (SCO) in Memphis. This growing service works with patients with learning-related vision problems, decreased vision secondary to eye disease, and vision problems resulting from brain injury.

He is the cosupervisor of the residency program in Pediatrics and Vision Therapy at SCO. This residency program has grown from one position to three in the past few years. Dr. Taub was instrumental in creating a new residency in Vision Therapy and Rehabilitation at SCO and assists private practitioners across the country in creating vision therapy residencies in their own offices.

Dr. Taub is a fellow in the College of Optometrists in Vision Development (COVD) and American Academy of Optometry. He served as the editor-in-chief of the Optometric Extension Program Foundation (OEPF) *Journal of Behavioral Optometry* and is the editor-in-chief of the new joint publication of OEPF, the COVD, and the Australasian College of Behavioural Optometrists, *Optometry and Visual Performance*. He is coeditor of the book *Visual Diagnosis and Care of the Patient with Special Needs*. He enjoys mentoring other optometrists through the process of becoming a fellow in COVD.

He is truly leaving a legacy in the field of vision therapy.

Jillian's Words about Marc

Dr. Taub teaches vision therapy. How awesome is that?

It is his goal to "tap into his students' passion and interest in vision therapy." He is an idol to me. I can't think of a better life than one where I could help patients and teach optometry students through my own experiences with vision therapy.

Dr. Taub keeps a thank you note from one of his patients on his office wall where he can see it every day. He truly wants to teach, help, and mentor others in his field. He is quick to offer assistance to schools, pediatricians, and psychologists who can't figure out what to do for a struggling child.

He said, "I know without vision therapy I would not be where I am today. To be able to work with and help kids who are just like I was is incredible. I can relate to each and every one of them in some way."

"I saw a kid yesterday who was so like me," he said. "Anything I can do to remove sight and vision as a barrier to learning, I will do. I don't want their vision to prevent their natural abilities from coming out or get in the way of them achieving their goals in life," he added.

Dr. Taub's son, Seth, is currently in vision therapy. Dr. Taub also has a niece who was born with amblyopia like me. She is in vision therapy for a second time. Unfortunately, in the middle of her first vision therapy sessions when she was a little girl, Dr. Taub and his family moved to another state. Her new optometrist was not a vision therapy specialist and he changed her lenses. Everything that her Uncle Marc had tried to do to help her was ruined. She is now in vision therapy again at the age of fourteen, and she is doing really well.

Seth is eight years old and he has both visual perceptual and tracking issues. His dad is not his vision therapist, which is probably a good thing. I don't know if I would have behaved in therapy if my dad had been my vision therapist. Seth gets to work with Dr. Paul Harris, who helps Dr. Taub's residents. Doctors Eric Weigel and Jen Idoni do the therapy. He likes vision therapy and never complains about going.

I asked Dr. Taub why so many vision problems seem to run in families. He told me that often "the apple doesn't fall far from the tree. The strengths and weaknesses of the parent will often manifest in the children."

If I am a mother someday, I will take my children to see an optometrist as soon as they are six months old. The American Optometric Association has a great program called InfantSee and optometrists all around America do free comprehensive eye exams for babies ages six to twelve months. I would not be surprised to have my own children in vision therapy someday.

I asked Dr. Taub if he kept in touch with Dr. Waldstreicher. He told me that they talk sometimes, and Dr. Taub thinks about his old doctor often. Dr. Waldstreicher once wrote in a letter to Marc, "In some small ways I believe that you are my legacy to optometry. Your accomplishments at this relative stage of your career make me glow with almost parental pride. Just as important have been your own personal experiences with vision therapy and the innate feeling that you have for it."

Dr. Taub, you really are my idol because I don't know whether I want to be an optometrist or a teacher . . . or maybe I could work for a foundation dedicated to helping others with vision problems. You've shown me how I could do it all and hopefully help others like you have.

John

"As a physical therapist, I have told people what to do for years. It's different when the shoe is on the other foot."

"The doctors think I've had five strokes," said John. "But I can really only tell you about three of them." John is only sixty-two years old.

The first stroke hit him in November 2009. He was working in the garage building a chair platform for one of his physical therapy patients. "All of a sudden, I had a buzzing sound in my head that turned into extreme dizziness. I got down on the ground, but couldn't get back up. I couldn't walk," he added.

"The doctors told me I'd had a stroke," he remembered. "I was basically kept sedated because every time I moved I started vomiting." After a few days in the hospital, John was moved to a rehabilitation hospital. He did daily sessions of occupational therapy and physical therapy as part of his rehab. "All of a sudden, I was the PT patient and not the physical therapist," he said. "I was in a wheelchair and not walking when I got there, but was lucky enough to walk with a cane when I left."

While at the rehabilitation hospital, a doctor suggested he might try vision therapy in conjunction with outpatient appointments for occupational and physical therapy.

"Even though I am a physical therapist, I didn't know anything about vision therapy. I would never have known about it without the rehabilitation doctor's referral," John said.

He scheduled an evaluation with Nancy Torgerson, Doctor of Optometry (OD), in Seattle.

"John was referred to me by an MD. Since the stroke, John noted double vision at near, blurred vision. He avoided reading and writing, computer work was difficult, and he had awkward and poor balance," said Dr. Torgerson.

"The evaluation revealed his eyes did not team together. He had limited ability to sustain over time. Not only was there a problem horizontally, but one eye also saw higher than the other eye. When a target was brought toward his eyes, he saw double out to nine inches. At near, his eyes told him things were farther than they truly were. At distance, objects appeared closer than they truly were," she added.

Dr. Torgerson said that on a visual field test, John was not able to see easily in superior gaze. His eye tracking movements were jerky, and his depth perception was poor. She recommended vision therapy for him.

"In vision therapy he worked diligently," said Dr. Torgerson. "He was able to see when his brain would suppress or ignore one eye's information as he did cheiroscopic tracings. Spatial localization was challenging at times. He fatigued easily."

"In nine months of vision therapy in the office and practicing activities at home, John regained the ability to team his eyes together and develop increased depth perception. Tracking became smoother," she added.

John worked for several months through the combination of OT/ PT/VT and gradually got better. He graduated from vision therapy.

"I was well enough to go back to work, but I worked thirty hours a week instead of forty." John was back on his feet, enjoying his job, and everything went well for the next two years.

"In November of 2011, two years after my first stroke, I was working when I felt a strange heaviness of my left leg and left arm," said John. It was another stroke. "It wasn't as bad as the first one, and I recovered fairly quickly and was able to go back to work," he added.

This time it was only seven months before John fell victim to his third stroke. Thinking back to June 2012, John said, "It was a horrible year. I had just gotten back to work after the last stroke when I lost my job. The company I had worked for as a physical therapist for years had to lay off a lot of people. And then I lost my wife. She was such a wonderful, wonderful person."

John ultimately found another job at a nursing home. "It was good to have a job and be back at work," he said. "I found that I would tire fairly easily, but I didn't worry about it too much," he added.

Two months after his wife passed away, while he was driving home from a visit to his son, John noticed that his mouth felt strange— as if it were full of marbles. He tried to talk, but his speech was slurred. He said he felt heaviness in his face, similar to the heaviness he had previously felt in his leg and arm.

"Obviously I should have pulled over and called 911, but I wasn't far and I just drove straight to the emergency room," he said.

His third stroke was the worst. "My vision was distorted, as if I had a fishbowl on my head. It was especially distorted when I got tired." He had balance problems and issues with his coordination.

"Realizing how much vision therapy had helped me the first time, my family doctor suggested that I talk to Dr. Torgerson again," John recalls. "I have been doing my second round of vision therapy for about six months and I am much better," he added. His struggles with visual distortion and balance are much improved.

According to Dr. Torgerson, "After this stroke, John described to me the same feeling—as though he were looking out from a fishbowl. He had more trouble with suppression of his right eye at near. At distance he could use both eyes together, but eye teaming was difficult at near.

The good news was that he did not lose all of his depth perception with this stroke."

Dr. Torgerson explains that John's vision was better than after his first stroke, but he had regressed from the time he graduated from vision therapy. He was now dizzy at the end of the day and generally more tired. John started vision therapy a second time.

"Again he was very diligent and had great awareness of his visual challenges. He struggled with right hand tremor, balance, and exhaustion," Dr. Torgerson shared. "After vision therapy sessions, he had to rest. Transition glasses were more bothersome when going on walks. But, with time, he has had amazing progress in tracking stereopsis, spatial awareness, central/peripheral awareness, vestibular/visual interaction, and visual memory. His goal to get back to work and drive truly was inspirational.

John had to stop driving after his stroke in June 2012, but recently he was cleared to drive. "I got my license," he said, almost like a giddy teenager. "I love to drive!" He has also been hired by a nursing home to do a little physical therapy consulting work. "I am so happy about that because I love my work."

John reports that "reading is easier, and when I spend a little time at the computer it is much easier. My 3D vision is better too.".

"Vision therapy really works. It's amazing how the brain can recover and relearn some things," John said. "It doesn't work automatically; you have to be steered, guided, and directed to heal in the right way."

John credits vision therapy, physical therapy, and occupational therapy for getting him back on his feet. "All three were very important for my recovery, to reach the point where I am now. All three disciplines helped to steer my recovery in the right direction," he said.

Jillian's Words about John

I've heard people talk about strokes, but I didn't really know what happens to your body or what it feels like to have one. I am so glad the doctor at the rehabilitation hospital told John about vision therapy. That should happen more. Some doctors have written to my mom and me since we wrote *Jillian's Story*. There are some doctors who don't believe in it, but there are also some who do. It makes me sad when parents say that their child's pediatrician strongly opposed vision therapy. In one case, a parent's insurance company simply needed approval from the pediatrician to cover vision therapy under that family's insurance plan. The doctor refused.

Why wouldn't a doctor want a family to look into any options that might be helpful? I know of several kids and teens who have gone through vision therapy, physical therapy, and occupational therapy at the same time, just like John did in recovering from his stroke. And, like John, they are much better now. If adults tell us kids to "keep an open mind," if people are open to the advances of new technology, then why can't physicians look at vision therapy with an open mind? I want to teach them about vision therapy and share with them what it can do and how much it can improve someone's life.

John said, "I think vision therapy helps people function at a better level than they could have without it." About vision therapy exercises, he said, "I have never left vision therapy without being exhausted. It's intensive and it's hard work. When I describe the exercises to people it sounds so simple, but it's truly a lot of work. It has really gotten to the source of my problems and it has helped me to be able to live my life."

I agree with John. That is why I call vision therapists "life-changers." John, I hope you never have another stroke. Thank you for sharing your story in hopes of helping others. I'm sorry you lost your wife, but I bet she would say you were wonderful too. I certainly think so!

Mikey

"I sat at the computer holding my son in my lap and typed into Google the word 'autism.'"
—Jim, Mikey's father

"It was like somebody flipped a switch," Jim said about his son. "Mikey was a normal baby boy until just before his first birthday."

Mikey's parents took him to his twelve month appointment with his pediatrician two days before he turned one year old. Mikey had the recommended immunizations at the appointment and later started running a fever.

"Right after that his personality changed," said Jim. "He stopped trying to talk and make sounds, and he wouldn't look you in the eye."

By the time Mikey was two years old, he still had not spoken a single word.

"We were obviously worried and looking for an answer," Jim recalled. They strongly suspected Mikey might be autistic.

Jim knew of an optometrist in his town who helped children with learning issues. He made an appointment and took Mikey to see Dr. Brad Habermehl. After an evaluation with Mikey, they discussed a way in which vision therapy might be able to help him.

"Mikey is the youngest patient I have ever had," said Ruth Villeneueve, his vision therapist. "He was only two years old."

Dr. Habermehl explains, "We discussed at length the best way to work with Mikey and decided to start with the Sensory Learning Program. Our office uses the Sensory Learning Program for many of our patients prior to beginning vision therapy. The program uses a gently moving table, modulated music, and different frequencies of light to open up the visual pathways and prepare our patients to respond more effectively to vision therapy."

Jim said, "I was amazed. They used lights and music and, although Mikey was a little upset at first, he would settle down."

Within two weeks of taking him to see Dr. Habermehl and Ruth, Mikey said his first words. "I was singing 'Row, Row, Row Your Boat' to him and he said, 'row, row, row.' I was amazed!" After completing the first part of Dr. Habermehl's program, it was time to start vision therapy.

"At first I just watched Mikey play," said Ruth. "Then I altered our program to make it work for a two year old. I didn't use our normal vision therapy room, but cleaned everything out of our waiting room so that it looked more like a family room. I put into the room only the things I wanted him to work with," she added.

The next step for Ruth was to figure out a way to use the toys he liked to play with in a way that would develop his visual skills and ultimately drive the development of language.

"Mikey loved to play with a penguin game that we had, so I decided to start working with that. I explained to him, in three to four word sentences, that he could only play with the penguin game when he wore the prism glasses. When he took the glasses off, I would temporarily put the game away. We repeated this process many times until eventually he left the glasses on and played with the game."

Ruth knew that as she worked with Mikey to improve his central vision, he would start talking more and more. Dr. Habermehl's evaluation showed that like many other children on the autism spectrum, Mikey avoided central gaze and attended to his periphery only. "This is why Mikey wouldn't look people in the eye," Ruth said.

"It makes sense when you think about the fact that as vision comes into the brain it travels through the language centers of the brain. We usually see improvements in a child's speech when they go through vision therapy," Ruth said.

Mikey's parents describe him as a very energetic child. But soon after starting vision therapy, they discovered that he would sit still for one thing. It was a show on Disney Channel called *Little Einsteins.*

"Mikey would sit motionless to watch that show and he would interact with it, answering questions and such," said Jim. "He wouldn't sit still for anything else."

When Mikey was three and a half, he started a special school program for autistic children. After a year and a half, a school administrator told his parents that Mikey no longer qualified to participate in their program.

"They said he had tested out of the program and that he was no longer autistic by their definition. They were very excited for Mikey, as they indicated that such a thing rarely happens," Jim said.

Mikey was able to start kindergarten in public school.

"I attribute all of it to vision therapy and the work that Ruth did with him. She just knew how to draw him out," said Jim.

Dr. Steve Gallop, optometrist and coauthor of *The Kingdom of Should,* believes that doctors should not put limits on anyone before starting vision therapy. He said, "Why wouldn't we offer to help when we have a process that is noninvasive, interactive, and, best of all, works?"

Dr. Gallop has seen vision therapy success with the majority of his patients on the autism spectrum. He collaborated on *The Kingdom of Should,* an audio story, with a friend who is a developmental music therapist.

"*The Kingdom of Should* provides information for parents about the field of Behavioral Optometry, which has a long history of success in improving the lives of children on the autism spectrum, yet remains unknown to the majority of parents seeking help for their children on the spectrum," Dr. Gallop said.

"Every child with developmental delays, learning differences, or any type of autism spectrum behaviors should be evaluated by a behavioral optometrist to assess visual development issues," he added.

Jillian's Words about Mikey

Mikey is now six years old and his parents are hopeful for his future. Jim said, "I think his experience with vision therapy has given him a chance to lead a more normal life."

Mikey no longer flaps his hands or walks on his toes. He plays fairly well with other kids and even has a best friend, Josh. He bowls on Saturday mornings and does really well.

His parents put him in a ten-week basketball program this past winter, and he loved to shoot the ball and became a very good shot. He didn't like to share the ball so much and didn't understand when the other kids played defense and wouldn't let him shoot.

He loves to dress up, especially as a superhero. He likes to wear a cape around the house and sometimes to school. He enjoys TV like most kids, especially cartoons or anything on Nick Junior.

Mikey is doing well in school, mostly having trouble when the teacher wants to redirect him to another lesson. He really likes his teacher, Mrs. O.

"He has a really great teacher who seems to understand him," said his dad, Jim. "There isn't a day that goes by where he doesn't mention her." At the last parent-teacher conference, Mikey got an excellent report. "His reading is at first grade level and he does very well in math and writing (as well as everything else). His teacher said he can get overwhelmed, so she tries not to challenge him beyond his comfort level.

Mikey's parents have referred another family from his school to vision therapy and he has done really well. Jim was also excited to share the success of another patient. He knows a girl who was told by her doctor that she would never ride a bike. When she started vision therapy, that was her goal. Recently, she raced in the BMX Great Lakes Nationals and came in third place.

"Mikey is a great example of how well early intervention worked thanks to his school and vision therapy," Jim said.

Dr. Neil Margolis is a developmental optometrist in the Chicago area. He often works with children who are "nonverbal, have developmental delays, or have multiple neurological diagnoses." He is a fellow of both the College of Optometrists in Vision Development and the American Academy of Optometry.

In an article in the June/July 2012 edition of *The Autism File* magazine, Dr. Margolis said, "For many children with autism, undeveloped and dysregulated vision can interfere with performance in several areas. Addressing these visual issues can lead to improvements in learning, attention, and even behavior."

Dr. Margolis added that it's important to understand whether vision is helping or interfering with a child's performance and development. "Optimizing the visual strategies and therapies available to us can yield significant benefits to children with autism." He said that having the parents involved is also the key.

He describes in the article how he can observe a child from a few feet away. He has a camera he can use that "screens for high refraction problems while taking a picture four feet away from the child." He can determine if the child needs glasses without getting too close and making them uncomfortable.

Dr. Margolis says that when he first meets a child, he usually dims the lights and encourages them to roam around the room while he talks to the parents. He often sits on the floor to make himself less intimidating and sometimes turns on a video. It depends on the child.

81

He said, "Nonverbal children often tell us, through their behaviors, what their problems are."

I hope Mikey has a great life. I hope he is happy. Thank you to his parents and to Dr. Habermehl and Ruth for taking great care of him. He was so young for vision therapy. But they didn't say that he was too young or that it couldn't be done. Instead, they put their heads together and found a way. Those are the kinds of adults that children, especially kids like Mikey, need on their side.

Christina

"Today I actually read for fun. I even own a Kindle."

Christina never realized that she had a vision problem. She thought everyone saw like she did.

"Growing up in New Jersey, I was mostly an A/B student," Christina said. "I may have earned a C in math or reading. I always did poor in math, but I was good at science, especially applied sciences," she added.

She got glasses for the first time in first or second grade, but she remembers that the prescription had to be changed often.

"I was an awful speller. Actually, I am a terrible speller to this day," she said. She recalls having to "study and study and study for spelling tests." Even with the extra study time, it was hard for her to make an A. "Writing a paragraph of a story was so hard. It would take hours for me to do writing assignments," she added.

In high school, Christina says homework took hours to complete. "The stress that builds with that is unbelievable," she said. She didn't play sports that required a ball, but enjoyed gymnastics and skiing.

She describes herself as "the kid in class who paid attention." She said she hated to read, but managed to do fairly well and graduated high school.

Christina went to the University of Pittsburgh in the late 1990s. After class one day, a professor pointed out that she had reversals in her writing. "I was surprised to see that I had written down the word "on" instead of "no," for example," she explained.

"My professor offered to send me over to see someone in the college of disabilities. They sent me for reading skills educational psych testing and it came back that I was 'learning disabled not otherwise specified.' They also said I had a mathematics disorder."

They told Christina she had a high IQ, but was not performing up to her potential. The private psychologist who administered the test suggested vision therapy. "That was how I met Dr. Len Press. I saw him when I was nineteen or twenty years old," she said.

Dr. Press said, "Christina was typical of college students that we work with who manage to get through elementary and high school with extraordinary effort. But in college the volume of work is too great, and the pace of assignments and testing is too fast and furious to compensate for poor visual skills simply by putting in more effort."

"In other words, the demand now exceeds the supply, and visual reserves are depleted very quickly. This is literally the case when a student has intermittent exotropia, or a tendency for one eye to drift outward excessively, which was Christina's primary diagnosis," Dr. Press shared.

"Given that it was fifteen years ago that Christina's college counselor suggested she look into a visual problem as a potential explanation for the discrepancy between Christina's potential and her performance, it was pretty enlightened thinking at the time," he added.

Christina said she remembers buying cassette tapes and recording herself reading chapters from a textbook. She would then listen to the tapes in her car to learn the material.

"I always wanted to be in a study group to have help," she recalled. She remembers taking breaks from studying. "I knew when my eyes were tired. I'd see words on top of words, and I knew I had to take a study break."

Thinking back to vision therapy, Christina said, "Vision therapy was difficult and I felt exhausted after the sessions. I remember driving home feeling so tired."

"Vision therapy was amazing. I remember the first time I saw a 3D picture. It opened up a whole new world for me. It was a little weird and I remember thinking, *Wow, so this is how other people see*," she shared.

Christina worked with Dr. Press throughout one college semester and over the summer.

"I cried when I realized that I wasn't stupid, but that I had a vision problem," she said. Christina knows she compensated for her vision problems over many years.

Dr. Press said, "It's very poignant hearing Christina's self-assessment after all these years. The instability of print that she describes, the visual fatigue, and the compromise in her depth perception were all indices of a binocular vision problem."

"Hopefully in sharing her story Christina will be helping guidance counselors and other professionals to give visual factors a consideration when there is significant discrepancy between intelligence and performance. Perhaps more importantly, it may spare students from questioning and self-doubt and give them the opportunity to improve their visual abilities just as Christina did," he added.

Jillian's Words about Christina

I know exactly how Christina felt. I used to think I was dumb or that other kids were born with a talent that I didn't have. So many children feel that way.

Christina successfully completed vision therapy and graduated from college. She has been a pediatric occupational therapist for eleven years. She said that more than half of the kids she has seen over the years have had vision problems. She refers parents to optometry when necessary and she currently has two of her patients in vision therapy.

Vision therapy has helped her not only personally, but also as an occupational therapist because of the vestibular system.

Dr. Press explained that "there is increasing recognition of the importance of interaction between visual and vestibular function in providing a stable visual environment."

"There is something called astronaut training, for example, which was introduced by two occupational therapists who work closely with optometrists, that incorporates exercises to help problems with visual and vestibular integration," Dr. Press said.

Vision therapy gave Christina the chance to pursue her career goals. Just think of the number of patients she would not have helped had her vision problems stopped her from graduating college and fulfilling her dreams.

Christina has joined a billiards league and, although she says she isn't the best player, she has fun. She also actually loves to read for pleasure now. She said, "I even own a Kindle."

I know that you will help many children through your work, Christina. I hope your story will be read by other occupational therapists, so that they might realize the benefit of vision therapy for their patients with vestibular problems.

Russell

"At age forty-two, I was the oldest student in my optometry school class."

Russell had worked for a Fortune 500 company in computer information systems for twenty years when he decided to pursue his passion for optometry.

"When I got married, my wife's exuberance and passion for her career made me rethink the decisions I had made about my own," Russell said. He spent a lot of time reflecting on his past and thinking about his future.

Russell was three years old when his pediatrician noticed he had "one bad eye." Russell's mother recalls that the doctor had Russ follow a pencil with his eyes. The doctor also noticed that Russell was high stepping when he walked, and his mother admitted that he had trouble judging where he was in relation to objects.

His primary care doctor referred Russell to an ophthalmologist, and Russ was diagnosed with strabismus and scheduled for surgery.

"I remember the eye surgery because it was such a traumatic experience," Russell said. "Back then, parents weren't allowed to stay overnight at the hospital with their children. I remember my mother telling me she'd see me after the surgery in the morning and I had a crying fit," he added.

After surgery, Russell recalls wearing glasses and starting limited patching when he was four or five years old. He wore a red lens cover over his eye. "They cut it out to fit my glasses and taped it there. Then they told me to watch television looking through the red lens cover," he said.

He remembers being the only kid in kindergarten who wore glasses and being teased about them. By elementary school, he did his best to avoid attention.

"I was a good student but super shy. I didn't want to play sports because I wasn't very coordinated. I remember faking injures just to keep the other kids from knowing I couldn't catch, throw, or hit a ball."

Russell had intermittent double vision at a distance, something he thought was normal for him. "I saw two teachers and everything was occasionally double at distance, but up close my vision was single. I was 100 percent certain that my problems with sports and eye-hand coordination were just me and never thought about it having anything to do with vision," he said.

Russell didn't struggle with learning; in fact, he loved to read. He was a straight-A student. It was not the academic part of school that troubled Russell, but the teasing and bullying from more athletically talented students. The stress of junior high and high school took its toll, leaving Russell with a stomach ulcer.

While many teenagers celebrate their sixteenth birthday by getting their driver's license, Russell found it stressful to sit behind the wheel. "When most of my classmates got their drivers' licenses, I got mine too because it was expected of me. Everyone was so excited about their new license, so I pretended I was excited too," he said.

Russell struggled with driving and didn't enjoy it at all. He was tentative and nervous because he had trouble judging distances. "It was an area of great stress for me," he recalled. "I didn't want to drive in reverse or parallel park. All I wanted to do was drive straight forward."

During his driving exam, he was instructed to reverse and park between two cars behind him. He finished parking and asked the instructor if he had done well. The driving instructor asked him to look to his left. When Russell looked left he realized how narrowly he had missed hitting the car next to him. "There was maybe five inches between that car and mine. It's a miracle I didn't hit it," he said.

Russell was instructed to try again and, much to his dismay, he parked the car just as closely to the car on his left as he had the first time. Finally he did an adequate job on the third try. "I asked the instructor if I had passed and he told me I did but that I wouldn't have passed if I'd hit that car."

He maintained his academic excellence throughout high school and graduated as salutatorian of his senior class. He went to Central Michigan University, where he majored in computer information systems.

"When I think of college I think of good memories, good friends, and good grades," said Russell. He was hired right out of college and worked for the same company for the next twenty years.

About a year into his career, Russell's company transferred him to Texas. He sought out a new optometrist. It was this optometrist who told him he had amblyopia.

"I grew up knowing I had a lazy eye, but don't recall hearing anyone call it amblyopia. I didn't understand the concept of my brain suppressing images. I thought it was just an eye turn issue," he said.

"My optometrist explained it to me and I found it all so interesting. About that same time I met a few new friends who were optometrists, and I wished that I had chosen that field as a career," Russell said.

Russell spent a long time reflecting on his career decision and his interest in optometry. "It was about that same time that my wife and I went on some mission trips with our church. We went to Mexico to help build homes," he said.

"I'm not a carpenter or much of a builder. I can't even hammer nails in a board, but I was able to help paint and do other tasks. I kept wishing I had a tangible skill and could be of more help to people in need," he added.

Russell decided to pursue optometry and went back to college at night while working during the day. After four years of working to meet the prerequisites, he was accepted at the State University of New York (SUNY) College of Optometry.

It was during his optometric education that Russell had an "a-ha" moment concerning his history of strabismus and amblyopia. He learned that his poor performance in sports, carpentry, driving, etc., was significantly influenced by his visual dysfunction. This revelation was profound and has greatly affected the direction of his optometric career.

At Russell's graduation, he was announced as the oldest graduate in SUNY history. He was forty-six years old.

Jillian's Words about Russell

After completing a residency in Family Practice/Ocular Disease, Dr. Russell Coates accepted a position as a Clinical Instructor at the Rosenberg School of Optometry, University of the Incarnate Word in San Antonio, Texas.

Dr. Coates didn't have vision therapy as a kid. Taping a red cover on a pair of glasses and telling someone to watch TV is not vision therapy. He first learned about it in optometry school. He had trouble learning to use a slit lamp, a piece of equipment optometrists use with every patient they see. It is helpful to have binocularity (both eyes working properly) to use a slit lamp.

Dr. Coates explained that, "Binocularity is advantageous in better perceiving certain anatomical changes, thereby helping the doctor in diagnosing."

He was sent to the vision therapy clinic to get help. As vision therapy restored his suppressed central vision, he began to have double vision at near. He struggled with intermittent double vision his whole life at distance, but he couldn't tolerate it at near.

He said, "Day in and day out my vision didn't bother me. I was used to it and it's all I had ever known. When I began to have double vision at near, I pulled away from vision therapy because I knew I'd never be able to do the reading necessary to learn and graduate from optometry school."

The doctor in charge of Dr. Russ's vision therapy told him that his prognosis was "guarded," and that there was a possibility of essentially having permanent near double vision. Dr. Russ explained that due to a few different factors such as his age and his primary reason for achieving binocularity being the use of a slit lamp, he agreed to take his doctor's advice and discontinue therapy.

We won't ever know if Dr. Russ could have pushed beyond double vision at near distance. It is possible that he could have because many people have done it, but there is also the chance he might have ended up with permanent double vision. I asked him about trying vision therapy now, but he believes he would have the same guarded prognosis and the same thing would likely happen.

"I learned so much about vision therapy and, although I decided to stop pursuing it, I realized how much it would have helped me when I was growing up," he said.

So, vision therapy didn't change Dr. Coates' life like it did mine. It changed his life in a different way: it made him determined and dedicated to help kids like himself and to teach optometry students so that they can help others.

It's not fair. If Russell had done vision therapy as a kid, his childhood might have been a happier experience. He endured bullying when vision therapy could have enhanced his coordination and sports performance. I think vision therapy would have helped him in so many ways that he could have avoided all the stress that made him ill.

I know that vision therapy works, but it wouldn't be fair of me to say that vision therapy works the same for every patient. I know of a lady in Utah who has seen vision therapy work for her son and daughter; it has also helped an adult friend of hers with amblyopia. But she has not achieved her vision therapy goal. I like to think of her as a work in progress and I hope someday she will find success.

Dr. Coates and I have similar goals in promoting vision therapy and I really admire him. He has taught me that it's never too late to set yourself on a new course in life and that you don't really have to graduate from vision therapy for it to change your life.

To Dr. Coates: you may have been bullied as a student, but now you are the teacher others need. You rock!

Kathy

*"I could have been back to work in two or three years if I had
received the care I needed."*

When her youngest son started first grade, Kathy decided to
go to law school. She was forty years old. But only two years into her
career, a head-on car crash altered her plans.

"I'd love to tell you about the accident, but I don't remember very
much," she said. She recalled that she was driving home from dropping
her daughter off at a Girl Scout meeting.

"I had let my son, who was eleven at the time, stay home
while I took her. My older son and husband had gone to a soccer
game, but I thought it would be only a few minutes," Kathy
shared.

She was close to her home when the accident happened. Someone
making a left turn apparently did not see her. At the crash site, she
faded in and out of consciousness but kept saying she needed to get
home to her son.

She was transported to the emergency room where she remembers
being asked repeatedly to name the presidents. "I was a political science
major, a lawyer. I seemed to remember enough going back to George
Washington to lead them to the conclusion that I was fine. But when I

insisted I had to get home to my son and they asked, 'What is your son's name?' I didn't know," she said.

Kathy finally managed to get in touch with a friend who promised to take care of her son and "I remember nothing after that. It was like, once I took care of that important task, my brain shut off."

Incredibly enough Kathy was released from the emergency room and her husband took her home, despite the fact that she fainted repeatedly while under observation. She was in horrible pain and thought perhaps her pelvis or back had been broken.

"I was in so much pain and confusion at home," she shared.

The following Monday, she saw her primary care doctor, who diagnosed her with a closed head injury. The doctor told Kathy she should heal for a while, and that she'd refer her to a neurologist in six weeks. Her doctor also referred her to physical therapy.

Upon finally seeing the neurologist, Kathy was sent to a variety of specialists. "He seemed to see all the broken pieces, which was helpful. The problem with a brain injury is that you can't figure out what you need. I knew something was wrong, but I didn't know what was wrong or why it was wrong," she explained.

One specialist on Kathy's referral list was a behavioral optometrist. "The neurologist and optometrist both noticed my eyes wandering everywhere, and I started vision therapy."

"Prior to the accident my vision was pretty darn good and I used to love to read," Kathy shared. "But with the brain injury I lost the ability to do so many things. I couldn't read. The words would jump around and I would get the worst headache."

"I couldn't cook, and I had truly enjoyed cooking. Grocery shopping was horrible. I would see cans bouncing around, and looking left and right as I walked down the aisle made me feel nauseated. My little boy would sit me down and take care of the shopping, pay the bill. It was an awful time," she added.

"I had to quit driving. I would get so lost every time I left the house. I would look, but not really see what was around me. It was really scary and I stopped driving."

The summer she started vision therapy, she asked her children's babysitter to drive her. "I always had to get someone to take me to vision therapy because I felt exhausted and horribly nauseated when I left," she said. "I doubt they know this, but I used to lie in the grass outside of the optometry clinic until my sixteen-year-old daughter came to get me," she said laughing.

"I could tell vision therapy was helping. I could read some, but I had trouble thinking what words meant," she said. Her headaches had diminished significantly.

"My company was so supportive and I tried to work. They let me try for months, but I didn't know what I was doing and I had to leave my job," she shared.

She and her husband of twenty-eight years got a divorce. "It was just beyond his capacity to deal with all of this," she said. "I no longer had the money to pay for vision therapy so I quit going. I also had no transportation. I tried continuing the home exercises, but it wasn't the same."

Kathy knew that vision therapy had worked for two of her children and she was convinced it would help her with her rehabilitation, but she was unable to continue. "Years went by and every day I either had a headache, was nauseated, or I was asleep," she said.

Although she couldn't work full-time at a law firm, she started volunteering as an advocate for people with traumatic brain injury in the state of Colorado. "I had a real need to help these people based on my own life," she said. She served on a brain injury task force.

She explained, "There was no care for people in our state, and insurance companies were turning down claims left and right. I was so horrified," she said. The goal of the task force was to help people with brain injuries to get benefits and for the state to develop an agency to help those affected.

After more than twenty years of efforts, Kathy is proud to report that there is now a Colorado Traumatic Brain Injury Trust Fund under the Division of Vocational Rehabilitation.

"Through my advocacy work over the years, I told people about my different therapies and they didn't get it. They seem to think that it takes a pill to fix a medical problem and if that doesn't work, then nothing else can fix it," she shared.

"I don't understand," she said. "These are smart people and I'm disappointed by their observation. Their narrowness of focus is doing people harm. I know without a doubt that I could have been back to work in two or three years if I had received the care I needed," she added.

She almost did not get that care at all, but, thanks to her brother, she continued to pursue the relief she needed.

"When my brother sold his business, he generously gave me the money to hire someone to help me on a daily basis. I immediately called Dr. Lynn Hellerstein for an appointment so that I could try vision therapy again after ten years," she said.

Kathy hired a "wonderful woman" to help her with cooking, errands, shopping, cleaning and medical appointments. "She saved me. Having her help turned my life around," she said.

Dr. Hellerstein saw Kathy in 2003. She said, "Kathy's symptoms included migraines, blurriness, fatigue, light sensitivity, dizziness, inability to read, and double vision, which worsened with fatigue."

Kathy was diagnosed with convergence insufficiency, hyperphoria (tendency for one eye to drift upward), visual spatial disturbance, and visual/vestibular problems. "All of these visual problems were related to her brain injury," Dr. Hellerstein said.

Dr. Hellerstein prescribed new glasses with a special tint to reduce light sensitivity. She recalled Kathy's comment about wearing her new glasses. "Kathy said, 'My eyes are happier.'" As part of Kathy's rehabilitative vision therapy, they used prisms, 3D equipment, eye movements, convergence/divergence activities, visual-spatial games, and visual processing activities.

They also incorporated Syntonics, which is the incorporation of specific frequencies of light applied through the eyes, which helps to correct visual disturbances at their source.

"I was so relieved to have a life and feel better," she said. "I remember being so excited to be able to follow the recipe on a box of muffins," she said.

Jillian's Words about Kathy

One of my latest vocabulary words in school was *resilient*. It means to be able to withstand or recover from difficult conditions. Well, that is Kathy.

Kathy did forty-four vision therapy sessions and she is now doing so well. Dr. Hellerstein said, "It has truly been a pleasure to be a part of Kathy's journey. Her persistence and self-motivation kept her moving through treatment. Although it took so many years to heal, she is one inspirational lady who shows it is never too late! Kathy is just one example of why I love what I do."

In addition to finding vision therapy, Kathy found help with Aston-Patterning. She described it as soft tissue work on her muscles. Aston-Patterning helped her realign her muscles and made her migraine headaches go away.

Kathy's vision therapy exercises and vestibular work have helped her to no longer have dizziness and nausea. She did quite a lot of visual memory work in vision therapy as well.

She can now drive, cook, and read. She does her own grocery shopping. She has enjoyed a little bit of traveling, has fun with wonderful friends, and loves to visit her kids.

She has put her twenty years of advocacy behind her and has been trained as a mediator. She is going to help people resolve their issues.

I'm sorry she had such an uphill battle in resolving her own issues, but she didn't give up despite the hard battle she had to fight.

I really admire Kathy, and I'm glad vision therapy has played a part in her recovery.

She said, "It has been helpful for my kids to see me trying and fighting. They know that setbacks are temporary and they feel empowered to keep going."

Nate

"I remember the entire experience of being the vision therapy patient. I think it makes me a better doctor."

It isn't unusual for adults to seek out vision therapy, but not many are students in optometry school when they realize they have a vision problem.

"I was always a good student but a slow reader," said Nate. "I did great in school, loved books, enjoyed reading. But I read very slowly."

Nate recalls getting glasses when he was about twelve years old. The optometrist mentioned in passing that Nate should have been able to see singular closer to his nose than he could.

"He said it along with other comments. He didn't make any recommendations for vision therapy or anything, and my family and I just let it go," Nate said.

Nate finished high school with good grades and went to the University of Florida. He describes his collegiate experience as a great one, but said he realizes now there were some areas where he could have done better.

"I studied a lot and never missed class. I hardly ever took notes, but I listened to everything the professors said. I couldn't just read a chapter from a textbook and get it."

After college, Nate pursued a career in optometry. He went to the Illinois College of Optometry in Chicago and that is where Nate realized he had a vision problem significant enough to stop him from pursuing his dream.

"I remember struggling with a lab exercise during the first year of optometry school. We were studying the near point of convergence. My lab partner could bring an object from in front of his face all the way to his nose without seeing double. I thought he was amazing!" I didn't realize that the norm is four inches from your nose and I was at twelve inches," he said.

Nate knew that when he was tired, he would begin to have double vision. "I just thought that was me, that it was normal," he said. "When I was studying and everything would start to go double, I just thought that was my sign that I was done for the night."

Nate describes himself as a morning person. He did most of his studying in the morning hours before his vision would trouble him.

"In my second year of optometry school, I couldn't compensate anymore. There were certain techniques we were learning in class and I couldn't do some of the procedures. I was worried that I wouldn't be able to be an optometrist. I was so frustrated."

Looking back, Nate recalls thinking that he had poor technique. "I still had not put it all together. I didn't realize I had a vision problem."

One of Nate's professors noticed his struggles using certain pieces of optometry equipment and suggested an eye exam.

"I was a textbook case of convergence insufficiency," he said with a small laugh.

Nate enrolled as a patient in the college's vision therapy clinic. He did weekly sessions with a therapist and several nights of home activities. He was a patient and a student at the same time.

"I experienced all the things then that my patients experience now," he said. He knows the ups and downs. He understands as they improve their vision. He knows the changes that come with vision therapy.

"After I finished vision therapy, I was super aware of space around people," he said. "Sometimes patients say that I might not get something that seems different to them, but I do. I get it."

Nate was finally able to do all the procedures and use all the equipment he needed to graduate from optometry school. "It is so funny, so ironic, that I struggled to (but finally did) pass the exams on optometry equipment that I use every single day as a doctor."

When asked what he thinks his life would be like today without vision therapy, at first he said, "I probably wouldn't be an optometrist." But then he thought for a second and replied, "Without vision therapy, I would not have given up, but I don't think I would have been as good of an optometrist. I would have probably felt frustrated and discouraged."

Nate says that his time in vision therapy has directly impacted the services he provides today. "It was about the time of me being in vision therapy that we started that rotation. I knew then that I wanted to offer vision therapy in my practice."

He thinks back to when he was a kid sometimes and thinks about the children he has helped. "When kids come to see me and they are extremely bright, I know they will find a way. But it wouldn't be anywhere near what their full potential could be."

Nate enjoys working with young sports enthusiasts as well. "Through vision therapy, we show athletes how they can take their good vision skills and get even better."

Jillian's Words about Nate

Dr. Nate is one of the first optometrists, besides my own, that I talked to about vision therapy. He sent me a list of questions right after *Jillian's Story* came out to interview me for an article he was writing. Now the shoe is on the other foot and I had the chance to ask him questions.

In addition to being a busy optometrist, Dr. Nate gives his time to help kids. He has published articles on how vision therapy can improve reading skills and taught many people about the importance of good vision. He gives of his time to offer school and community vision screenings and has traveled to Nicaragua as a member of Volunteers in Optometric Service to Humanity. He has helped examine and distribute glasses to thousands of people.

He is the past chairman of the social media committee for the College of Optometrists in Vision Development. I had a really fun experience with Dr. Nate in 2011 as I helped launch the COVD "Visions of Hope" Video Contest. I put together a fun salute to Harry Potter to demonstrate how vision therapy worked like magic for me. The contest led many people to share their own stories of vision therapy success. You can watch several of the videos and find information about the Visions of Hope contest at www.COVD.org under the "Children's Vision and Learning Month" tab.

It's amazing that Dr. Nate discovered his vision problem while in optometry school. Vision therapy has changed his life, not only because it allowed him to finish school and go on to become the optometrist he is today, but also just think of all he lives he has changed through his office and volunteer efforts. My mom calls that the domino effect.

Dr. Nate, you are so inspiring. I think the domino effect you have on people goes beyond help offered and lives changed. I am lucky and proud to be one of the "dominoes" in your life. You may not have been my personal optometrist, but you'll always be one that I admire very much.

Teri

"The doctor said I'd never be who I once was."

It was a perfectly normal morning. Teri had wrapped up her daily routine and was about to leave for work. She took two steps toward the door and suddenly the room started to spin.

"I was so dizzy that I couldn't even walk. I had to crawl to the bathroom, where I started vomiting," she said.

Her husband, Skip, came home from work to take her to the emergency room. She was horribly dehydrated from severe vomiting, and the hospital staff started her on IV fluids.

"One of my eyes was circling clockwise and the other, counterclockwise. I had to keep my eyes closed," Teri said. The doctors thought she was possibly having a stroke.

As a speech pathologist, Teri worked at Tacoma General Hospital and knew many of the staff members. "As I went into the room for an MRI, a coworker said, 'All of your tests are STAT. What's going on, Teri?' and I told him I had no idea," she recalled.

The emergency room gave her medicine to control the vomiting and told her to contact her primary care doctor if she still felt ill the next day. "All the medicine did was stop the vomiting; the room was still spinning," Teri said. She also had a roaring sound in her left ear and was struggling to hear out of it. "I went to see my doctor and he referred me to a neurologist," Teri shared.

Three days after her emergency room visit, Teri met with her neurologist. "He ruled out stroke and multiple sclerosis. He said I had polyneuritis and that it was brought on by Guillain-Barre Syndrome (GBS)," Teri shared.

The neurologist explained that GBS is a virus that can cause cranial peripheral nerve inflammation. The syndrome can affect people in different ways. She told the neurologist that, in addition to constant vertigo, she was having double vision. "He gave me an eye patch to wear," she recalled.

Another three days went by with no improvement. Teri decided to seek the advice of Dr. Curt Baxstrom, an optometrist who specializes in vision therapy.

Teri said, "In my work I see patients ages eight and up in rehab for balance and vision. I have personally referred several patients to vision therapy and have seen significant gains. I knew of Dr. Baxstrom's success in treating patients through vision therapy."

Dr. Baxstrom said that Teri had a paresis of one of her eye muscles, and he gave her prism in her glasses.

"The double vision went away immediately and I could see," Teri said excitedly. "He suggested I wear a visor because the light was killing me. He taught me how to stabilize myself, how to balance, so I could have some function in my daily life." Teri started seeing Dr. Baxstrom weekly for vision therapy.

"My routine was to get up for two hours, go back to bed for four hours, get up for two more and so on," Teri said. She had worked for twenty-three years on the rehabilitation team at the hospital as a speech pathologist. She once worked nine to twelve hours a day and, once a month, she would work fifteen days straight without a day off. Now she would lie in bed almost all day.

Teri shared that she also went to an ear, nose, and throat specialist who ran tests on her. "He said there was no cure and that I would never be who I once was," she recalled. She was fifty years old.

Two months later the vertigo was gone, but Teri experienced a chronic feeling of movement similar to being on a boat. Walking was extremely difficult, but with the vision therapy skills Dr. Baxstrom had given her, Teri learned to cope. "I learned how to increase the motor signal to make up for the improper signal I was getting from my eyes. One activity was simply rolling my fingers. Another helped me to stabilize my head so I could walk straight," she said.

"Each time I saw Dr. Baxstrom, he gave me new exercises to improve both my balance and my vision," she said. He suggested Teri get a walking stick and start out walking five steps with the stick in her left hand and then five steps with it in her right.

This exercise was intended to synchronize Teri's vision and motor systems, "I did this when I was awake and out of bed during those two hour intervals, and I could walk about six hundred steps a day," Teri shared.

By this time, she was able to move her head slightly from side to side and focus on a specific target to help stabilize herself. She reported to Dr. Baxstrom that her fatigue was significantly better. She was able to occasionally cook a meal and do a load of laundry.

Teri said wearing a visor under florescent lights significantly helped her fatigue. She started physical therapy, where she began with traditional balance exercises and later moved to neurostructural integration techniques.

"Everything Dr. Baxstrom suggested was so helpful," she said. "I was trapped by people who didn't understand how drastically my life had changed." She remembers being invited to dinner with friends, but she didn't know how she could get through the day, much less going out to dinner.

"I remember going to a restaurant and having to hold on to chairs and tables because everything was spinning and I was watching the clock. I knew I would have a horrible week if I pushed myself too far."

"Even my doctor's office didn't understand what I was going through. I went for an allergy test and I was kept waiting for three hours," she said. "I kept turning off the lights in the room and the nurse would come in and turn them back on when all I could tolerate was natural or florescent light while wearing a visor," Teri shared. Her doctor had three emergency patients come in who needed to be served ahead of her scheduled appointment time.

"I told the nurse that I had to leave and she told me I couldn't leave until I saw the doctor," Teri said. Teri's simple allergy test turned into a week of recovery time on her end.

Jillian's Words about Teri

Teri said, "My life is significantly improved because of the skilled therapy provided by Dr. Curt Baxstrom."

Teri said that vision therapy never made her feel sick or caused her any setbacks. She reported that Dr. Baxstrom decreased the diopters (the measurement of prism) in her lenses a little at a time until her vision returned to baseline. He didn't simply use vision therapy exercises; he got creative to find answers for Teri. He searched for and addressed the underlying causes of her vertigo.

Teri remembers using a Brock String and doing exercises with a ball on a string. Teri said, "At first when the ball would make a half-circle toward me, I would fall over, but now I can stay on my feet and catch it!" She did vision therapy for two years and still does some of the exercises, which help her with daily activities.

Teri said that thanks to her husband, she feels pretty normal now. He retired from his job to take over things at home. He does most of the cooking, cleaning, and errands.

It has been four years since Teri found out she had polyneuritis. Today, she is driving and back at work. She has worked up from a schedule of seeing four patients (with a nap between the first and last two) to working seven to eight hours a day. Just this year she has started reading, watching television, and listening to music again. She is now walking well enough to use a treadmill and can walk for one to two miles. She only needs the walking stick if she is going more than a few blocks.

Teri has good days and bad days. "I can be very functional, but my life has to be structured," she said. She kept a log throughout her struggle, which she shared with me. If you look at the log, you can see a pattern of a good day, like Thanksgiving, followed by two or three days of rest. One of the days that caught my attention was Easter. Teri wrote:

Saturday, April 3: Excellent 7:00 a.m.–1:00 p.m. Lots of cooking for Easter. Family arrived in the p.m., up late.

Sunday, April 4: Family, no rest, did well.

April 5–6: Unable to work. On couch all day. Overdid it!

I think Teri is one smart, brave lady! She has, with the help of Dr. Baxstrom, forged a new path in her life. She has kept enough great information about herself to understand what works best for her. She knows it's not a good idea to have more than one appointment a week, so if she needs to see the dentist, a haircut will have to wait.

Teri, I am glad vision therapy has changed your life for the better. It is obvious to me that your struggles brought out your strong, fighting spirit. There is nothing wrong with knowing your limitations, especially with your sweet husband to help you. If anyone ever tells you again that you'll never be who you once were, I say smack them with your walking stick and head straight out their door. Walk on!

Mary Ellen

"I know what the families suffering through a loved one's brain injury are going through because I went through it too."

Mary Ellen is tremendously proud of her son, Jeremy. After all, his story is nothing short of miraculous and his life is tremendously inspirational. But it is Mary Ellen's story as Jeremy's mother and a former special education teacher that we found unforgettable.

Jeremy's birth was long and dramatic. Mary Ellen was in labor with Jeremy for two and a half days. After birth, doctors checked him over quite thoroughly before sending him home to his loving parents and siblings. Jeremy never crawled but took off running one day at the age of nine months. It would be an understatement to say he was an active child.

Mary Ellen said, "When Jeremy was two or three years old, I was troubled by the fact that he couldn't follow simple directions." For example, one time Mary Ellen and Jeremy were getting ready to go run some errands. Mary Ellen simply asked Jeremy to go upstairs and get his shoes. "I found him sitting on the stairs with a puzzled look on his face, and I repeated the instructions to him again."

A few minutes later Mary Ellen found Jeremy in his room, crying. He was scratching at the floor, banging his head, and repeating to himself, "not know, not know." She got down on the floor, took him into her arms and cried with him.

Jeremy had trouble with speaking and always scrambled words in his sentences. "I always explained to those around him what he was trying to say," Mary Ellen said.

One day when Jeremy was trying to ride his tricycle, Mary Ellen was heartbroken to hear the neighbor children teasing him. "He fell off his trike and they laughed. He started falling off and acting goofy just to make them laugh and it upset me so much," she said.

Mary Ellen took Jeremy to see a pediatric neurologist, who conducted several tests over a period of weeks. They concluded that Jeremy had severe brain damage from his difficult birth. "When I heard the doctor say, 'Your son has brain damage,' I sat there shaking my head." The doctors showed her the x-ray of Jeremy's brain and pointed out the damaged areas, but Mary Ellen kept thinking it couldn't be true. The doctor told her she was in denial and suggested she seek counseling.

The doctors also diagnosed Jeremy with ADHD and told Mary Ellen they doubted he would pass the cognitive age of five years old. She recalled, "They said there was nothing we could do for him and that he would always need someone to take care of him."

Although doctors suggested that Jeremy's parents not enroll him in preschool, they did it anyway. "Two months after he started, the school said he was not socially mature enough to be there," Mary Ellen shared.

A year later, Mary Ellen decided to pursue schooling again and made an appointment with the school psychologist. "He said they could try putting him into school, but that he didn't want to share Jeremy's information with his new teacher right away. He suggested they wait and see what she had to say after Jeremy had been in her class for a while," Mary Ellen shared.

"The school psychologist came with me to meet with Jeremy's teacher when conferences rolled around and she said she was not having any problems with him, but she suggested he needed speech therapy," Mary Ellen said. The psychologist then informed Jeremy's teacher of his brain damage, and she was very surprised. "His teacher said she never would have guessed," Mary Ellen recalled.

But the elementary years were not easy on Jeremy, and he was tremendously stressed about school. When he was in the fourth grade, Jeremy's parents were told that his disability was too severe and he could not be educated. It was for this reason that they chose to homeschool Jeremy and his siblings.

Mary Ellen said, "We used a specific curriculum and kept everything very structured." She began to look for activities she could do with Jeremy to help him with learning. It was during her research that she found some information about vision, learning, vestibular, and sensory integration.

Jeremy started doing pencil pushups, figure eights, cross crawls, and snow angels on the floor. Mary Ellen had him try jumping jacks, crawling, and anything else she could come up with to help him focus and simulate learning.

Jeremy's doctor recommended Ritalin, but Mary Ellen decided to try a special diet of all clean and natural foods and continue the visual and vestibular activities she had discovered. She had never heard of vision therapy, and none of Jeremy's doctors had ever mentioned it.

Mary Ellen recalls how things started to change. The entire family went to Florida on a vacation to see family and visit Disney World. Jeremy seemed very relaxed and calm. He loved Disney World and all the rides. He came home talking about taking more vacations in the future.

Thinking back, Mary Ellen wondered what it was about the spinning rides and roller coasters that Jeremy loved and why it seemed his behavior changed so much after the trip. After talking to experts, she now believes it's possible that the vestibular stimulation of the rides at Disney World had something to do with Jeremy's cognitive improvement.

That Christmas, Mary Ellen's brothers and sisters noticed a major difference in Jeremy. Jeremy's parents had made the decision never to tell anyone, including family, about his brain damage because they didn't want Jeremy to be treated differently. Mary Ellen says a simple comment from her brother really surprised her. "He said, 'What did you do with your kids, trade them in for new ones?' and I ran upstairs crying," she said.

"We told them the truth about Jeremy that night and they were shocked. They couldn't believe we had never told them," she said. "They truly noticed a difference in Jeremy that Christmas, when he was fourteen, and the changes just kept coming," she added.

Jeremy went to public high school when he was a sophomore. His dad had taught him how to play basketball when he was younger and he was a very good player. Jeremy tried out for the high school basketball team and the coach made him a starter.

Academically, he was placed in the school's advanced program and graduated from high school with a scholarship offer to a two-year community college. Mary Ellen said, "I was bawling when he graduated because my hope was that he could just get through school."

Jillian's Words about Mary Ellen

Mary Ellen is proud to report that Jeremy went on to complete his bachelor's and master's degrees. He now has a PhD in business and marketing. He is a professor at Florida State College in Jacksonville, Florida. Jeremy has led a very normal adulthood. In addition to his career, he also has a son; Mary Ellen is a proud grandmother.

After Jeremy's high school graduation, Mary Ellen worked as a special education teacher for seven years. One Sunday at a church function, a local optometrist sat with her. She began to tell him a little about Jeremy and, the more they talked, the more he was convinced that Mary Ellen would make a wonderful vision therapist.

Mary Ellen shared, "At first I said no because I was a little burned out with all the years in special education, but I went to see what he did in his office and I knew I had to work there." Mary Ellen realized that the special exercises she had created during Jeremy's homeschooling years were some common techniques used in vision therapy.

Today Mary Ellen works mostly with brain-injured, autistic, and special needs patients at Dr. Rick Graebe's office in the Children's Vision and Learning Center of Versailles, Kentucky. She said, "My work is very rewarding. I know what the families suffering through a loved one's brain injury are going through because I went through it too."

She said, "Patients with brain injuries, whether organic or traumatic, do make progress, but at a slower rate. Their success comes one small step at a time, so patience is very important, for them and for their families."

One of Mary Ellen's first patients had suffered a traumatic brain injury in a car accident. R. C., who was referred by a rehab center, could not walk without the help of a walker and talked with great difficulty. After just three months of vision therapy, the rehab center was so impressed with R. C.'s vestibular improvement that they came to Mary Ellen's office to see what she'd done to make such a difference.

Mary Ellen said, "Actually, R. C. was in a wheelchair when he started vision therapy, but graduated to a walker and then to a four point cane. His speech improved slightly and I understand he's continuing with some speech therapy. His stability increased and his dizziness decreased significantly. He also no longer experienced diplopia (double vision) and his eye-hand coordination improved."

Hannah, another of Mary Ellen's patients, had four eye muscle surgeries prior to trying vision therapy. During her second round of vision therapy, Hannah began to see in 3D for the first time in her life. She stated that before vision therapy, snow looked like it was coming down in front of a window. But after therapy, it was like she was actually in a snow globe with the snow falling all around her.

Mary Ellen is now a Certified Paraoptometric Assistant and a Certified Optometric Vision Therapist. Her story is unique in our book because neither she nor Jeremy experienced vision therapy as a patient. She has changed the lives of many of the patients in Dr. Graebe's office with a strong, personal understanding of their challenges because of her role as Jeremy's mother and teacher.

You can read more about Jeremy and Mary Ellen in the Optometric Extension Program Foundation's *Journal of Behavioral Optometry*, Volume 23/2012, www.OEPF.org. In this article, Mary Ellen shared that while in high school, Jeremy was involved in Distributive Education Clubs of America (DECA). He was selected as the most outstanding DECA student in the county and was featured in the local newspaper. Mary Ellen sent the newspaper article to Jeremy's doctor and the psychologist who originally diagnosed him with brain damage and ADHD.

"They said it was impossible for the child they saw to accomplish that," Mary Ellen said. "They asked what we had done. When I told them, they were more than amazed," she added.

Mary Ellen says her strong faith in God gave her the strength and determination to never give up on Jeremy. I wish Jeremy's parents had found out about vision therapy when he was little. I hope stories like Jeremy's will help doctors to understand that we can't give up on people.

Many parents have written to my mom and me, and they are angry and upset that they were either never told about vision therapy or told it doesn't work. Isn't it better to try something than to live with the regret that you didn't?

Thanks to Jeremy for sharing his story. Mary Ellen, thank you for reminding us to never give up, to try new ideas, and to go our own way.

I think your work as a vision therapist will change the lives of many people with special needs.

Joshua

"We thought Joshua would be living with us for the rest of his life."
—Michele, Joshua's mother

At twenty-two months of age, Joshua had strabismus surgery on both eyes. He was missing developmental milestones and was still not talking by age two.

"Joshua started speech therapy when he was two. He has and continues to attend weekly speech therapy provided by our county," his mother, Michele said. "His speech was not good when he was little. I could understand him, but others looked to me to translate," she added.

In addition to his speech challenges, Michele worried about his developmental delays. She recalled that Joshua had a friend in his playgroup who had been diagnosed with autism. "It made me wonder about Joshua," she said.

Between September 2008 and May 2009, Joshua participated in the Study to Explore Early Development (SEED), sponsored by the Kennedy Krieger Institute (KKI) and Johns Hopkins. The study concluded that Joshua was delayed in all areas.

"Also during this time, Joshua had several ear infections. The ENT described to us that Joshua had been hearing as if he were underwater for those entire four years," Michele said. She thought his speech problems were naturally the result of his limited hearing.

In January 2010, Joshua was seen at KKI in the Center for Development and Learning (CDL) office. Michele shared, "The nurse practitioner took Joshua to various departments for assessments. He went to the speech department and, upon further testing, it was discovered that he had dysarthria (oral motor issues)."

"He can move his tongue up and down, but not side to side," Michele explained. "Despite his many years of working with a specialist, through his school and outside therapy, Joshua had made little headway in speech therapy.

Michele said that during the summer of 2009, Joshua was given a test for sensory integration and processing through the school and it came back that he was below average on everything. "In addition to speech therapy, the county added in occupational therapy for fine and gross motor skills.

"We didn't know what to do or how to handle this, so we hired a special advocate to help us navigate with the school system. He was seen at KKI for various developmental issues and testing throughout the entire school year," she added.

During the summer between pre-k and kindergarten, Joshua's school reevaluated his Individualized Education Plan (IEP). "At the same time we took him to a neurobehavioral specialist for diagnosis. We were told that he had Pervasive Development Disorder--Not Otherwise Specified (PDD-NOS), or moderate autism. The doctor said he would be living with us for the rest of his life and that Joshua would not ever be able to hold down a job and function normally in society," said Michele.

Michele recalls that Joshua first wore glasses at the age of four-and-a-half. The same ophthalmologist who had performed the strabismus surgery prescribed his lenses. "We had a fifty-seven inch big screen television and Joshua would sit about two inches from it to watch a show," she shared. "When I asked the ophthalmologist about it, he said that Joshua would grow out of it. Those were his words," she said.

During kindergarten, Joshua started seeing an occupational therapist, Julie, who worked with him at school and in her private practice over the summer.

Michele shared that when Joshua was in first grade, Julie performed the Sensory Integration and Praxis Text (SIPT) on Joshua. "The test results showed us that Joshua needed vision therapy. I had never heard of it, and I thought he was already doing so many different therapies that we couldn't add anything else into the mix."

But Michele took Julie's advice to heart and called Joshua's ophthalmologist to ask his opinion of vision therapy. "I told him that I needed Joshua's records and that we were considering vision therapy," she said. "He said we shouldn't waste our money. He said they are all quacks and to not do it."

But Michele did not stop there. She called on many other specialists and did her own investigation into vision therapy. "It was confusing. Our occupational therapist was saying to do vision therapy and our ophthalmologist was saying not to do it. After talking to several people, including doctors, we decided that we could leave no stone unturned. I did not fully understand vision therapy until the first meeting with Dr. Marsha Benshir and she put it all into perspective for me."

Dr. Benshir said that Joshua's initial examination was different from any testing he had previously. "This was the first time that anyone really tried to find out how he was seeing," she said.

"His acuity was not well developed but more important than that was that he could not localize in space," Dr. Benshir explained. "This means that not only was it hard for him to know what he was seeing, but he had no idea where he was seeing it. This affected his perception of himself as well as his ability to interact with his environment. His interpersonal (play) skills had been impacted, and it added an additional level of frustration to everything he tried to do," she added.

Michele recalled that, upon completing Josh's comprehensive eye exam, Dr. Benshir asked her if the ophthalmologist who performed Joshua's strabismus surgery at twenty-two months had suggested vision therapy. "My answer was no," she said. "He never mentioned it and if he had, we would have done it. I told Dr. Benshir that I thought once the surgery was performed it would make the eyes go straight and that his vision and sight would fall into place. I had no idea that it didn't work that way."

Dr. Benshir explained that when looking at a target, Joshua not only had difficulty bringing detail into focus but could not determine if he was seeing one or two of the same thing.

"Usually it was two objects that moved and overlapped. This caused a great deal of stress for him and interfered with information processing," Dr. Benshir said.

"His poor ability to use his eyes together had been masked by the surgery that aligned his eyes, but the surgery did not stimulate the neurological processing of information from the two eyes together," she explained. This misinformation was more of an impairment for Joshua than if he had been using just one eye at a time.

Michele said, "Dr. Benshir also pointed out that Joshua was seeing two moms and not one. That's why he was constantly turning his head when he looked at me—he only wanted to see one mommy. I never knew that!"

Jillian's Words about Joshua

Joshua is now nine years old and has been recently diagnosed with high-functioning autism. He is doing well in school. He is very loving and sweet to people. He will play with other kids although he sometimes prefers to play alone.

Joshua didn't like vision therapy all that much at first. He went every Wednesday morning before school. At first his mom stayed with him in the room because it was all new and a little scary. She remembers him complaining at first, asking, *When is this over? Are we done yet? Can we go home?* Joshua would get frustrated at times because the activity wasn't something he enjoyed or he "just plain old didn't want to do it." Michele credits his vision therapist, Sam, for getting Joshua to do what he needed to do.

He enjoyed doing exercises such as a ball toss and memory match game. Dr. Benshir said, "Although there were many tests and some of them were too hard for him to perform, Joshua really tried and maintained attention through many difficult tasks."

"He had obvious problems with eye alignment, ocular motor skills were poorly developed, and his visual processing had not really started to develop. This means that in addition to poor fixation and tracking, he had no depth perception, poor form and figure-ground perception, poor spatial skills, poor directionality, underdeveloped eye-hand coordination, and poor visual-auditory integration," she added.

Dr. Benshir told me, "Think about it: Joshua had not developed good auditory or visual processing skills, which means that all information input and learning would be impeded!"

It was super important that Joshua cooperate with vision therapy exercises. The prize box proved to be a great motivator.

Joshua said, "Dr. Benshir's office had a prize box and I could choose one prize and two little pieces of candy if I were well behaved and did my therapy well that day."

I'm told Dr. Benshir's office also does a monthly prize drawing for kids who do their vision therapy homework and bring their folder back each week. Josh won the drawing once and got a $10 gift card to Pizza Hut.

That's brilliant. I'm telling you, the prize box is a huge incentive for kids. I would have been an angel for my vision therapist, Lindsey, if a pizza were on the line.

Josh says that his life has changed because he can see correctly. He can play games and cards, enjoy his iPad, ride his bike, and watch TV while sitting on the couch instead of two inches in front of the screen. He likes baseball and basketball more than ever because now he can hit the ball and make baskets. He says he can think better and his speech has improved. His grades are much better in school.

Joshua likes school. He said, "I enjoy video games, Wii Mario Kart and Tanks, watching *Scooby-Doo* shows and the *Star Wars* movies, *Thomas the Train* (shows and playing with them), John Deere equipment, books, and I absolutely love legos!"

Joshua has changed in so many ways since he was diagnosed with Pervasive Developmental Disorder—Not Otherwise Specified (PDD-NOS), moderate autism. Michele said, "The doctor that diagnosed him said that Joshua would not be able to be on his own as an adult because he would not be able to function properly in society. We thought Joshua would be living with us, his parents, for the rest of his life."

When asked about her son now, Michele enthusiastically replied, "Joshua has evolved into this wonderful human being full of surprises and life. He has grown in so many ways I can't even begin to count."

Joshua is riding a bike and not running into things. His mother says he is not repetitive like he used to be with questions. "Sometimes he would repeat the questions maybe seventy or more times before stopping," she said. "It is like the wheels are constantly running and not getting trapped in a hole in a road like before," she added.

"He can now look at me, eye to eye, without turning his head and see one of me," Michele said. "He will learn to drive a car, graduate from high school, and go on to bigger and better things because the sky is wide open for him now. He can explore whatever he chooses as a career and maybe one day marry and have children."

I am thrilled for Joshua and the life he has ahead of him. My mom and I always say that vision therapy is more emotional than clinical. At least, it feels that way. I think this is true for Joshua's family.

Josh, I am a huge Wii Mario Kart fan and I'd love to challenge you to a game or two sometime. I also have a Scooby-Doo stuffed animal and some of those movies on DVD. I know your mom won't be anxious to see you move out on your own someday, but she'll be truly happy to know that you can. Good luck with everything in your life. I think you have many fun and fantastic days ahead of you.

Toni

"I had panic attacks while driving my car."

She was afraid to drive. So afraid, in fact, that Toni put off starting a recommended vision therapy program for an entire year.

"I had vertigo and dizziness while driving in the car and that led to panic attacks," Toni said. "There I was, a thirty-three-year-old woman, sitting on the side of the road trying to calm down. I tried soothing music and even bought a lavender pillow because lavender supposedly has soothing qualities," she said.

Nothing worked. Her doctor put her on Xanax for the panic attacks. She went to see an ear, nose, and throat specialist for vertigo testing. She saw a cardiologist in case her problem was high blood pressure.

"It was actually the ENT doctor that suggested I needed to get my vision checked," Toni said. "I thought since I wore contacts and had regular check-ups that I was 20/20."

As a child, Toni recalled having vision problems. She had an eye turn and remembered her mother doing vision exercises with her.

During her visits to many different specialists, Toni went to see an ophthalmologist. "He gave me a prism to hold in front of my eye when

I read. He suggested doing it for about twenty minutes every night," she described. "That didn't work."

Then her ophthalmologist suggested eye drops for an eye spasm. "That didn't work either. Nothing worked," she said.

Toni said it was during a phone conversation with her mother that she found a possible answer.

"My mom said when I was little I did vision exercises, vision therapy. So I looked it up on the Internet. That is how I found Dr. Nate.

"In my first appointment with him, he asked me so many different questions, used different methods. He told me that I had myopia (nearsightedness), astigmatism, convergence insufficiency, and accommodative infacility. I was so relieved to know there was something he could do to help me," she recalled.

But Toni didn't go to vision therapy for another twelve months.

"It was a forty minute drive to Dr. Nate's office. My anxiety was so high and I was just too terrified to drive to his office."

"Everyone kept saying that I needed to get the anxiety under control before I could go to vision therapy, but the truth is that I had to get my vision corrected in order to get the anxiety under control."

Dr. Nate said, "I was very happy Toni came back because many adults really want vision therapy but then either have health or family issues and never get to it, despite our best efforts. Toni was very motivated from the beginning and that had a lot to do with her success."

Toni said, "I remember feeling nauseated a few times early on in vision therapy. It didn't make me feel stressed. Vision therapy was actually fun!"

"My favorite exercises were the Brock String, Eccentric Circles and Barrel Card because they were easy to do and I could do them almost anywhere," she said. "I really can't think of any exercise that I didn't like at all; most of them are kind of like little games, and I was happy something was working," she recalled.

"I graduated from vision therapy after only five months, one month earlier than Dr. Nate thought I would. I was a maniac about doing the home exercises and did twice as much as my vision therapist said to do," Toni added.

"Vision therapy was not a long process for me and it's the most amazing thing," she said.

The best part to Toni was that she was back to driving without panic attacks in only six weeks. "I was actually driving the speed limit," she added with a laugh.

In addition to the relief from anxiety, Toni noticed other changes after vision therapy. "I go for walks every day and I have for a long time. One day I noticed a bush while on my walk and I realized it looked different and amazing."

She thought she must have developed some sort of "super vision," but then it occurred to her that *this* was how things were supposed to look.

Toni reports that she doesn't take medication as much as she used to and doesn't get vertigo or dizziness or a feeling of car sickness any longer.

"I can watch action movies now, whereas they used to make me nauseated. I can see 3D without the blur. It has helped me at work as well. It was getting harder and harder to see my spreadsheets no matter how large of a font I used. The columns no longer blur together," she said.

Toni said her husband describes her as a different person. He used to complain that she was a horrible backseat driver and would insist that she close her eyes and rest her seat all the way back when they were in the car together.

"I was constantly smacking the dashboard and asking him if he could see okay. I was second guessing him and other drivers because I thought they saw things like I did," Toni shared.

Jillian's Words about Toni

Toni has her confidence back. She is trying things she always wanted to try. She said that reading is fun again.

It is not unusual for kids to have panic attacks and anxiety due to vision problems. Dr. Nate said the same is true for adults. He said, "Vision problems do generally cause stress, which affects every person differently. With children I think this most commonly shows up in the form of test anxiety or anxiety while reading. Adults generally have more stress in their life and have dealt with it for longer periods."

Toni said she felt like she was in a permanent state of headache prior to vision therapy. Now they are gone.

I am so happy that she has her life back. I can relate to Toni because we both went out after vision therapy to try new things. I think it was natural for me because I was a kid, but I think it took guts for Toni to put her troubles behind her and be adventurous as an adult.

One of the new things that Toni has started doing since vision therapy is equestrian horseback riding. Can you believe that this woman, with major anxiety issues and panic attacks while riding in a car, is now riding on the back of a horse? And not just any horse—a horse that leaps into the air and jumps big hurdles. That is so cool!

Toni recently entered her first horse show and won three blue ribbons. She was named the champion of her division.

I went roller skating for the first time a few days ago. My parents never let me try it when I was little with my vision problems. I know now that it would have been terrifying. Can you imagine trying to skate with double vision, no depth perception, and little peripheral vision? It used to make me feel so jumpy and on edge walking in crowds of people who seemed to suddenly appear out of nowhere from beside me. Having that happen while moving on skates would have freaked me out.

I'm glad I tried skating. I didn't enjoy falling all the time and moving with no control, and I can't say that I'm a huge fan of having wheels on my feet, but at least I tried it.

I want to snow ski. I want to try snowboarding. I'd like to parachute from an airplane and soar in a hot air balloon. And, thanks to Toni, I think I'd like to try equestrian riding.

Toni describes her vision therapy experience as "going from old-fashioned tube television to high definition TV." She told her physician about vision therapy. Toni said, "My doctor was very happy to hear that it worked and said she would keep it in mind for future patients with the same complaints that I had."

"Vision therapy definitely works. It worked so well for me," Toni shared.

Me too, Toni. I love your spirit and hope we both have many fun adventures in life. Keep trying new things and have fun. Remember, no fear!

Beanie

"I could never read to my kids."

She couldn't read above a fourth grade level until she was fifty-five years old. "The day I found out I had a vision problem was the first day in my life that I didn't feel like a dummy," Beanie said.

She recalled the torture of school. "They held me back in first grade and I had remedial reading in second grade." Third and fourth grade were horrible years. "I wanted to leap out of my chair and run outside whenever it was my turn to read out loud in class," she said.

Beanie remembered struggling to finish work in class and having to stay inside with the teacher if she needed extra time or special help. "I missed recess many times."

Her effort and hands-on classes helped her get through school. She did receive her diploma. "The thing I remember most about high school was how much I wanted to help with the school newspaper. I couldn't read or write very well, but I volunteered to staple all the papers together. That was my job," she said.

Beanie said her options were very limited when she got out of high school. "I had been babysitting and working as a waitress and I liked that, but I knew I needed a better job. I thought I'd go to beauty school, but when they handed me a stack of books, I knew I couldn't do it. I was so sad," she remembered.

Although the textbooks intimidated her, Beanie still gave beauty school a try. She thought she could learn by watching. But one day when the instructor asked the students to cut one inch of hair off of a mannequin, Beanie made an inaccurate judgment of length and snipped off three inches. "The instructor held it up in front of the class as an example of how not to do it. It embarrassed me so much and I quit."

After getting married, Beanie found a job at Grede Foundries. She and her husband started their family and she was a stay-at-home mother until her son was three years old. She then went back to work as a waitress for four years before taking a job in a local factory making golf tees.

"I remember my son telling me when he was five years old that his teacher read way better than me," Beanie shared. She worried and wondered how she would be able to help her children with their homework.

"I decided to go to a GED class, thinking it might help me with reading. They told me I could only read at a fourth grade level. I tried really hard for two months, trying my best to work on reading, but I realized it was pointless. I said to my husband, 'I'm not going to be able to read to the kids,'" she said.

Thanks to a couple of friends, Beanie decided to pursue a home-based business. "I thought it sounded so great. I loved the idea, but when I went to the orientation meeting, they said, 'The more you read, the better you'll get and the more you'll understand it.' I started crying and I thought, *I can't do this either.*"

Her friends rallied around her and insisted that they would help her be successful. Beanie has run her home-based business for many years.

"One day I decided to try going to job service to see if they might have a program for adults who couldn't read," Beanie said. "They told me I would have to see a social worker and a psychologist. I met with the social worker and took time off work to meet with the psychologist. After the testing, he told me that I was severely dyslexic and asked me how I had managed to get through school," she recalled.

"I told him through my best effort and hands-on courses like home economics. I started to cry and he asked me if it came as a shock to me. I told him no and asked him what I could do about it. He said, 'That is the hard part at your age.' He walked away and I never saw him again." Beanie was fifty-two years old.

She lost her job at the factory when operations were moved to China. She said her employer paid to remediate her and she worked with another reading specialist two hours a day, four days a week.

"I remember being asked if I'd had a vision perception test. I was sent to see an optometrist. That was the first day in my life that I didn't feel like a dummy," she said.

Beanie was evaluated by Developmental Optometrist Dr. Heidi Johnson at Superior Eye Health and Vision Therapy Center in Marquette, Michigan. Dr. Johnson confirmed a problem with visual processing and perception as well as convergence insufficiency.

Dr. Johnson said, "When Beanie tried to look close, she had trouble converging or pulling her eyes in. Her eyes did not work as a team."

Dr. Johnson explained this was the reason for Beanie's symptoms of eye aches, trouble tracking, and words moving or jumbling on the page. No wonder she had difficulty concentrating and understanding what she saw!

She explained that Beanie also had poor depth perception, a common sign of binocular eye teaming problems.

"Even though Beanie had many eye exams throughout the years, she never had some of these simple visual tests. She was happy to know there was a reason for her difficulties and that there was something she could do about it," she added. Dr. Johnson designed a program of vision therapy for Beanie.

"I was going nowhere in life and I decided I had to try vision therapy," Beanie said. She drove 180 miles round trip once a week for six months.

Dr. Johnson said that Beanie was skeptical about the visual activities she had to do in therapy. "At her second session with vision therapist, Jada Christensen, she questioned everything," said Dr. Johnson. "After watching a swinging ball and catching it between her fingertips, she exclaimed, 'And doing *this* will help me read?' So Jada explained how important it is to make accurate spatial judgments and for the eyes and hands to work together," she added.

Beanie practiced four to five different visual activities every day at home. Her first progress check with Dr. Johnson was after eight weeks of therapy. Already, her depth perception was improving. Her eyes were learning to be a team. Dr. Johnson measured her convergence and was happy to report the therapy was working. "Beanie continued therapy, building block patterns and practicing seeing them flipped or turned. Now she began to understand she was developing her 'mind's eye.'" Changes were happening in Beanie's brain! She began to feel more comfortable looking close. Her confidence grew."

Beanie's reading was retested. With her vision work, her reading improved from low comprehension with a fourth grade reading level to faster speed and comprehension at the sixth grade level in just a few short months. Dr. Johnson said that these results were quicker than anything Beanie had tried before. "She enjoyed the activities even though some of them were hard. She had to play tic-tac-toe without paper, just using her visual memory to plan her moves. This helped her learn to visualize or see pictures in her head. Soon, she noticed she was able to recognize more words without sounding them out."

At her next progress check, Dr. Johnson retested her visual processing and perception. Her visual memory had improved from the second percentile to the twenty-fifth percentile. Visual figure-ground perception improved from the seventh percentile to the fifty-third percentile. Visual closure, which is the brain's ability to "fill in the blanks" (like in playing Wheel-of-Fortune) improved from the first percentile to the sixteenth percentile.

"Beanie was starting to see and understand like everyone else," Dr. Johnson said.

"My reading and writing have improved so much," Beanie shared. "I noticed recently that I could write on a straight line and make addresses look straight on an envelope," she added.

Jillian's Words about Beanie

I saved the first email I ever got from Beanie because it really touched me. She wrote:

Jillian,

I am so proud of you. I was never able to read to my kids or above a 4th grade level until I was 55. I am now 60 and just had a kids book published called "Never Give Up . . . Beanie's Story." It is truly my story.

Keep up your great work!

Beanie

Beanie is amazing. She went through so many hard years in her life and never quit trying to find an answer to her reading problems. She continued to look for help and I'm glad she finally found it.

She was inspired to never give up by a friend's daughter who had a brain tumor. "She told me that someday I would read and that I would succeed and it made me want to try," Beanie shared.

Beanie shared that she had coffee every Wednesday with a friend who encouraged her to write a book. So, being Beanie, she found a class about entrepreneurship. She started writing. At her son's wedding, she met one of her new in-laws who is a freelance writer and together they finished her book. She found a wonderful illustrator who helped her book become a reality.

"My husband and kids are so proud of me," she said. She now visits schools and shares her message with children. "I usually asked the students how many of them have parents or grandparents that read to you. And then I tell them I could never read to my kids."

Beanie has led many children to vision therapy. Her book mentions vision therapy. She said in her book, "Beanie realized for the first time that she was smart after all, she just needed special help because of the way she sees."

Beanie said her optometrist also introduced her to ChromaGen lenses for people battling dyslexia. She went from reading seventy-seven words per minute to ninety-nine words per minute. She explained that it has something to do with how the light flows and hits the brain.

Beanie, I think it's wonderful that you've written your story to help other kids avoid the struggles you had in life. You can now read to your grandchildren. Thank you for being a brave example of why it's important to never give up in life.

Beanie's book is available at www.BeanieLeffler.com.

Zach

"His suicide comments had become too frequent. He was only seven years old."

Zach always looked happy to see his mother when she picked him up after school. But every day was the same routine. He would be happy for a few moments and then start a fight with his little brother during the ride home. Once in the house, things would escalate further with tantrums and screaming.

"He would usually run and hide in my bathroom or closet and scream. It got to the point that I would go to the other side of the house until he could calm himself down. When I tried to talk to him, he would react even worse," said Zach's mother, Janna.

"I could see him hiding quietly, but, as soon as he saw me, he would start screaming," she said. This was a daily occurrence for many months. "Parenting books started piling up on my nightstand. I blamed myself," she added.

Zach would often tell his mother that he wanted to kill himself, and he once tried to choke himself in front of her. "You are never prepared for something like that," she said.

"The psychologist said that Zach did it out of anger to hurt me," Janna shared. "But I later came to believe she was wrong."

As a pediatrician, Janna had an extra close eye on her children's health. She was aware that Zach crawled as he should and that he started walking at fourteen months old. Before the age of two, Zach began to exhibit some "odd behavior."

"Zach was always very quirky. He had an obsession with things that spin. He liked to flip his little toy cars over and watch the wheels spin. He played with handheld fans and adored analog clocks. His absolutely favorite thing to do was to sit and watch the clothes spin in our frontloading washing machine," Janna said. He was very attached to his mom and dad, but had no attachment to stuffed animals or a blanket. "He did not go through terrible twos," said Janna.

She recalled taking Zach to see a specialist for testing. "He was not diagnosed with autism spectrum disorder, but I think a different psychologist might have diagnosed him as such." Zach was diagnosed with Attention Deficit Disorder (ADD), inattentive type.

When Zach was two-and-a-half, Janna and her husband, also a doctor, began to notice that Zach crossed his eyes when looking at them at the dinner table. Janna took him to see an ophthalmologist right away.

"I was worried it was a medical issue because of some of the cases I've seen, but we were told he had intermittent accomodative esotropia due to excessive farsightedness. I was told at that first visit that he was lucky. We had caught it early, and he didn't have amblyopia. But the doctor wasn't sure if he was getting full cooperation from Zach and we continued to monitor him closely over the coming months," Janna shared.

After moving from Maryland to Arkansas, Janna took Zach to see a new pediatric ophthalmologist who said Zach was maybe 20/30 in his left eye but indicated no problems. At age five, just three weeks after a routine follow up appointment with his pediatric ophthalmologist, an optometrist volunteering at Zach's preschool sent home a note that he had a serious vision problem and to please follow up with an optometrist.

"I was so mad! We had just seen the doctor and he said everything was fine with Zach's vision," Janna said.

Janna began to wonder if Zach was somehow cheating in his eye exams. Based on her medical background, she had chosen to take him to an ophthalmologist and not an optometrist, but she started having second thoughts.

She decided to seek the opinion of another ophthalmologist, who diagnosed Zach with amblyopia and instructed Zach's parents to begin patching his weak eye two hours a day. He wore a patch for three years.

During that visit, Janna remembers explaining some of Zach's history. "I told the doctor it took Zach forever to get his homework done, that he just couldn't stay on task. I told him that Zach complained daily of a mild headache. The doctor did not connect those dots for me."

"Second grade was the worst. Zach was in serious emotional distress," Janna said. Homework that should have taken twenty minutes at most was a two- to three-hour nightmare.

"Zach could tell the most creative stories, but he couldn't write them down. Every single afternoon he would start screaming and I knew it was because home was his safe place and he could let out all of his frustration," Janna shared. "But to hear my small child say, 'Please bring me a gun that is loaded with a bullet to shoot myself in the head,' was just more than I could take," she cried.

A friend of Janna's had taken her child to vision therapy and to see a doctor in New York who specialized in ADD, dyslexia, and learning disorders. "We didn't talk specifically about her child's diagnosis or what vision therapy was. She told me it had helped her child, but she didn't seem to know very much about it. She seemed to think the cause of most of her child's problems was a poorly functioning vestibular system," Janna shared.

"My son was seen every few months for five years by an opthalmologist. I reasoned that it couldn't possibly be an undiagnosed vision problem," she added.

Not even considering vision therapy, she and her husband decided to take Zach to the specialist in New York. He put Zach on an over-the-counter medication called meclizine, which is used to treat nausea, vomiting, and dizziness caused by motion sickness.

"I had been told to ignore Zach's outbursts and tantrums and to not let Zach know he was getting to me, but I honestly couldn't hold it together," Janna shared.

Coming home from the trip to New York, Janna and Zach had a chance encounter that Janna believes saved Zach's life. "We met a nice man on the plane named Jerry. He is the one that told me about vision therapy." Jerry followed up after the trip by sending Janna an email link to an article about convergence insufficiency.

"I didn't understand developmental optometry. I thought an optometrist would be limited to refraction and then refer us back to ophthalmology. I thought I was just saving us a step in that process," Janna said.

"I was aware of a little bit of a turf battle between ophthalmology and optometry, but I thought whatever politics existed were based on surgical procedures performed by optometrists," Janna said. "Most medical doctors don't know what optometrists do. I didn't," she added.

Janna immediately emailed Zach's ophthalmologist about vision therapy. "He said Zach did not have convergence insufficiency and that vision therapy did not work," she said. But she couldn't stop thinking that "it just made sense." Janna began to research vision therapy on her own.

She said, "The meclizine helped Zach feel happier, but he was still having tremendous learning challenges. I decided to make an appointment with an optometrist in North Little Rock. I was astonished. I took Zach for an eye exam that told me more about his problems than any other exam—ever."

She recalls watching Zach go through an exercise while wearing 3D glasses where he was asked to put the plus sign on the center of the circle. "He was off by six inches," Janna said. "He saw double and his optometrist put him in bifocals to keep his eyes from crossing in the near range," Janna shared.

Zach also had vestibular problems, which explained so much about his interest in things that spin. According to Curt Baxstrom, M.A., O.D., a Fellow of the American Academy of Optometry and the College of Optometrists in Vision Development, "Some children crave visual stimulation. It can be calming."

Dr. Baxstrom explained that our vestibular system incorporates input from our eyes, ears and body. He said, "It's auditory for hearing, vestibular for movement of the head, eyes for central and peripheral input, and your body for motor sensory input. If you modify input to any of them, the rest are simultaneously affected as well. With vision therapy, we incorporate the bilateral systems of motor, vestibular, and visual to help patients reach their highest possible potential."

Janna said, "When Zach got his bifocals, he looked out the car window on the drive home and said that nothing really looked that different, but when we got inside the house he pulled a book out of his backpack and said, 'Momma, this book has *letters* in it!'" Zach said letters used to look like "hairy, gray blobs."

From that day forward, Zach never mentioned killing himself again.

Jillian's Words about Zach

Zach's story makes me want to cry. In fact, I have cried both sad and happy tears for Zach. I remember the day we first received an email from Zach's mother. My mom kept choking up as she tried to read the note out loud to me, my dad and sister. We were all in tears hearing about how much Zach had suffered as a little boy.

Vision therapy really changed Zach's life. In fact, his mom would tell you that, in conjunction with occupational therapy, it saved Zach's life. Zach liked going to vision therapy. He did many of the same exercises that I did. He also used a computer program and did exercises at home.

He graduated from vision therapy after only eight months. Homework is no longer a nightmare and he reads for fun. His mother was surprised one day to find him reading to his little brother.

Like me, Zach was given contacts to wear at a young age. I saved an email that he sent me. He wrote:

My name is Zach and I'm 7 years old. I have heard about your story. I do vision therapy just like you. I almost went blind in my left eye, but I wore a patch on my right eye and did vision therapy, and my left eye got better. Now I decided to wear contacts. I got them yesterday. So far, I can only wear them for 2 hours a day. I attached pictures of me with glasses and with contacts. I look kind of nice with glasses, but I like the way I look better with contacts. Contacts aren't so bad because once you get used to them, you forget that they are in your eye.

Zach is such a cute kid! He is now ten years old and doing really well. His mother has been studying about primitive reflexes, the vestibular system, and visual processing. She wants to help train other doctors about this.

Zach used to say about himself, "I'm so stupid," but his mom hasn't heard his say that since he did vision therapy. Now he will tell you he is smart, and he has confidence and self-esteem. He has lots of friends, fits into the crowd, and sticks up for kids that get bullied.

He enjoys reading and learning. His favorite books are from the *Guardians of Ga'Hoole* series. He enjoys science and plays the piano and violin. He got roller skates for Christmas and has taught himself to skate. He loves *Harry Potter*, which is another thing we have in common.

I asked his mother why some medical doctors don't believe in vision therapy. She said, "One of Zach's ophthalmologists showed me a text book that he used in medical school. There are only two sentences in the book about vision therapy that basically say vision therapy does not work and that it could be harmful to those who pursue it."

That's just wrong. I don't think it's right to base opinions solely on a textbook. My elementary and middle school science textbooks taught me that Pluto is a planet, but it hasn't been one since 2006 when it was downgraded to a dwarf planet by the International Astronomical Union (IAU). A *National Geographic* news article said, "This decision will force textbooks to be rewritten."

Textbooks can be wrong. They can also be rewritten.

To my friend, Zach, enjoy being a kid! I think you are a lot like Harry Potter. You both had battles to fight and villains to overcome.

To Dr. Janna, they say never to underestimate the power of a mother. I am in awe of your strength, courage, and determination, not only in helping Zach, but as a pediatrician willing to educate your peers and the world about the benefits of vision therapy. You will change many, many lives.

Resources

Web

Optometric Extension Program Foundation (OEPF)
www.OEPF.org

College of Optometrists in Vision Development (COVD)
www.COVD.org

Neuro-Optometric Rehabilitation Association (NORA)
www.NORA.cc

American Optometric Association (AOA)
www.AOA.org

InfantSEE
www.InfantSee.org

Australasian College of Behavioural Optometrists (ACBO)
www.ACBO.org.au

British Association of Behavioural Optometrists (BABO)
www.BABO.co.uk

Parents Active for Vision Education (PAVE)
www.PaveVision.org

Books and More

Jillian's Story: How Vision Therapy Changed My Daughter's Life, by Robin Benoit with Jillian Benoit
www.JilliansStory.com

See it! Say it! Do it! (book and workbook), by Dr. Lynn Hellerstein
www.LynnHellerstein.com

Fixing My Gaze, by Dr. Sue Barry
www.FixingMyGaze.com
www.StereoSue.com

The Kingdom of Should, by Joan Raina, Joe Romano, and Steven J. Gallop
www.KingdomOfShould.com

Looking Differently at Nearsightedness and Myopia, by Steven J. Gallop
(Available through OEPF and at Dr. Gallop's website,
www.GallopIntoVision.com)

Endless Journey: A Head-Trauma Victim's Remarkable Rehabilitation,
by Janet Stumbo, MD
(Available through OEPF)

Visual Diagnosis and Care of the Patient with Special Needs, by Marc B. Taub, OD; Mary Bartuccio, OD; and Dominick M. Maino, OD
(Available through OEPF)

How Behavioral Optometry Can Unlock Your Child's Potential: Identifying and Overcoming Blocks to Concentration, Self-Esteem and School Success with Vision Therapy, by Joel Warshowsky
(Available through OEPF)

The Suddenly Successful Student and Friends, by Hazel Dawkins; Ellis Edelman, OD; and Constantine Forkiotis, OD
(Available from Amazon.com and through OEPF)

Vision Therapy Success Stories
www.VisionTherapyStories.org

About the Authors

Robin Benoit

Robin is proud to be an advocate for vision therapy and comprehensive eye exams. This is her second book. Her first book, *Jillian's Story: How Vision Therapy Changed My Daughter's Life,* sold thousands of copies worldwide and helped countless children and adults find proper vision care.

A graduate of Oklahoma State University with a degree in journalism and public relations, Robin was honored to serve as a national officer for her sorority, Phi Mu. Robin began her career in the nonprofit field before moving on to advertising agency and corporate communications positions. She put her career on hold when Jillian was diagnosed with amblyopia to become a homeschool teacher to her daughters. She describes these three challenging years as the most rewarding to her as a parent.

Robin loves to travel, a passion that began when she was a college student during her Semester at Sea in 1984. She now resides in Fort Collins, Colorado, with her husband, Brian, her daughters, Annelise and Jillian, and their dog, Boomer. Her email is Robin@JilliansStory.com.

Jillian Benoit

The positive impact that vision therapy has had on Jillian's quality of life is almost indescribable. Without it, she would not be able to live the life she now leads.

Jillian is a freshman honor roll student at Fossil Ridge High School in Fort Collins, Colorado. She is a member of the marching band, in which she plays the clarinet, and is involved in a number of school clubs and activities. She is also very active in public speaking and advocacy efforts. Along with her mother, Jillian received the Making Vision Therapy Visible Award in 2011 from the College of Optometrists in Vision Development for "Outstanding Contributions to Public Awareness of Optometric Vision Therapy and Developmental Vision Care."

Now fourteen years old, Jillian is the coauthor of two books about vision therapy. She very much wants to help children and adults who are living with vision challenges. Please contact her at Jillian@JilliansStory.com should you know of a child needing a supportive pen pal.